THE 90-DAY WORKOUT JOURNAL FOR MEN

DAILY MOTIVATION TO TRACK YOUR FOOD & EXERCISE GOALS

VANCE HINDS

ROCKRIDGE PRESS

Interior and Cover Designer: Michael Cook
Art Producer: Sara Feinstein
Editors: Andrea Leptinsky and Rachelle Cihonski
Production Editor: Ruth Sakata Corley

All illustrations used under license from Shutterstock.com

ISBN: Print 978-1-64876-220-8

R0

This Journal Belongs to:

_____

FOREWORD

If you're reading this book, odds are you've already decided to change your life for the better. Congratulations! Now, if you're scratching your head as to why a three-time professional wrestling champion and WWE Hall of Famer is writing this foreword, well, that's a bit of a longer story that you might want to research more on your own. Go ahead, I'll wait . . .

When I first saw the video that Vance Hinds, weighing in at 475 pounds, posted on Twitter promising to do something about his health, I thought to myself, "That's pretty bold to put it out there for everyone to see!"

And when I offered my support to him, I didn't realize that he had NO IDEA who I was and why I was coming forward to help. The cool thing about Vance, though, was that he had decided to say yes to literally any idea that might help him get closer to his goal. He had an open mind, even when the outcome was very uncertain. He very well may have succeeded without my help, but I still like to think I played a small part in him losing nearly 200 pounds in a single year.

Let's be clear, though: As they say in any weight-loss commercial you see on TV, "These results are not typical." But are they possible? Vance is living proof that through hard work, consistency, and a structured plan, such change is possible (even if you're starting at 475 pounds). Vance's mind-blowing transformation has been shared tens of millions of times, which in turn has inspired many others to take that first giant step.

As important as the first step is, it's only going to get you so far. I'm so proud of Vance for what he's accomplished, but *even prouder* that, in this journal, he is sharing the things he learned along the way to impact other people's lives. This journal really can be game-changing if you use it and put in the work.

So c'mon! Get going! I believe in YOU . . . do you?

—Diamond Dallas Page (DDP), *WWE Hall of Famer, and founder and CEO of DDP Yoga*

INTRODUCTION

Over the last three years, I've lost 228 pounds and 80 inches; I've eaten 1,150 eggs and 237 salads; I've biked 1,110 miles, swum 95 miles, and completed 726 DDP Yoga sessions. I started my weight-loss journey at the age of 52, weighing 475 pounds, with two guiding principles: commit to yes, and post everything online. These two principles profoundly changed my life.

My mentor, retired professional wrestling superstar Diamond Dallas Page, created DDP Yoga, a combination of traditional yoga moves, old school calisthenics, and dynamic resistance. I know how many of Dallas's workouts I completed because I kept a journal of all my stats on my fitness journey—not a formal diary, but a compilation of phone notes, pictures, and posts.

Through this process, I learned the value of journaling—not just tracking your food, but tracking everything: exercises, progress pictures, measurements, and mental health. There are as many diets and exercise programs as there are grains of sand on a beach. No one size fits all. Each of us is unique, with different desires, capabilities, and opportunities. Lasting change depends on finding a plan that suits you; creating that plan begins with knowledge; and knowledge comes from journaling.

No existing journal accommodates the entirety of the diverse fitness landscape, so when I was presented with the opportunity to create my own journal, I jumped at the chance. I wanted to create the book I never had on my fitness journey: the most complete and versatile workout journal for men. No matter your path to better health, this journal will guide you by tracking your nutrients, exercises, and progress. As Dallas would say, with the knowledge you record in this journal, "You can own your life."

HOW TO USE THIS BOOK

There is no single correct way to use this book. Mold it to fit your specific situation. If you eat carnivore, fast daily, and run ultramarathons, this journal is for you. If you eat vegan, meditate, and do Vinyasa yoga, this journal is for you. If you eat dirty keto, power lift, and compete in no-gi Brazilian jujitsu tournaments, this journal is for you. When you buy this journal, treat it like the brim of a new ball cap: Start molding immediately to fit your needs!

The journal contains three parts: Establish Goals, Make Progress, and Review Results. In part 1, you'll establish your baseline, set your goals, and create your fitness plan. In part 2, you'll document your daily activities. This section is your molding ground. You can record information about your exercises, macronutrient intake, water intake, and sleep habits. A star-ranking system provides a quick reference for your performance. In part 3, you'll analyze the data, tweak your fitness plan, and plot your next move. Also included is a Resources section of additional tools and learning guides that helped me on my weight-loss journey.

You may be wondering: Why 90 days? Two reasons. First: In 2009, a study published in the *European Journal of Social Psychology* investigating the process of habit-forming in everyday life found that, on average, it takes 66 days to form a habit. Sticking to journaling for 90 days should create a lasting practice that will benefit you for the rest of your life. Second: You eat an elephant one bite at a time. In 90 days, you can eat anything. Get to molding and eating!

ESTABLISH GOALS

In November of 2017, I weighed 475 pounds. Diagnosed with a bad heart and two bad knees, I could not get the knee surgeries I needed unless I lost 175 pounds. I saw no light at the end of the tunnel. But I promise you: Life can be different. In 2019, I completed 20 triathlon-style events, including a 100-mile bike ride, an Olympic triathlon, and a 2.4-mile open water swim. Change in life starts with small goals and small habits. That's where part 1 comes in! It's time to put pen to paper to set your baseline and your goals. Let's get you started.

SETTING INTENTIONS

As you get started on your workout journey, look ahead to the goals you hope to achieve. What would make you feel more agile, healthier, and happier in 90 days?

First Intention: Outer Journey

Your first goal should be something you really want to do. Set a date and time for the event and make it public. Whether it is walking a 5K, lifting 300 pounds, or competing in a grappling tournament, schedule it and shout it from the mountaintop!

Second Intention: Inner Journey

Your next goal should be something that would make you feel good inside. Think about how you'll feel when you can fit into old clothes, when you lose a certain amount of weight, or when you can tie your shoes. Take a close look at yourself, and write down what you want to change. This goal is your private goal.

THE MEASUREMENT LOGS

Welcome to the first of many measurement sections. The Measurement Logs are your scorecard, the home for your stats. Using a measuring tape, measure and record the parts of your body spotlighted in the chart on page 5, along with your body mass index (BMI), resting metabolic rate (RMR), and resting heart rate (RHR).

Your **BMI** is your weight (in kilograms) divided by the square of your height (in meters). High BMI can indicate the presence of a high amount of body fat, but BMI should not be relied on by itself as a measure of your health. The CDC hosts a BMI calculator on its website (see Resources, page 115) that also provides information on your BMI weight status category.

Your **RMR** is the energy your body needs to function while you're at rest. It usually accounts for the largest portion of an individual's overall energy requirements. RMR is typically measured after 15 minutes of rest. Basal metabolic rate (BMR), a similar value, is measured under more stringent conditions: after the subject has performed an overnight fast, hasn't exercised for 24 hours, and is in a calm and restful state. MyFitnessPal hosts a BMR calculator on its website (see Resources, page 115) that you can use to quickly estimate your RMR/BMR.

Your **RHR** is the number of times your heart beats per minute while you're at rest. Generally, the lower your RHR, the healthier and stronger your heart is. It's easy to measure your heart rate manually: Place your fingers on the inside of your wrist, count your pulse for 30 seconds, and multiple that number by 2 to produce your heart rate in beats per minute.

We are all different. BMI, RMR, and RHR are useful tools for tracking your weight-loss journey, but remember that your "normal" may differ from someone else's. Most important is to record, record, record, record! As your journey progresses, the information you write in these logs will become invaluable.

STARTING MEASUREMENTS LOG: BODY CHECK-IN

DATE:_____

NECK	
CHEST	
SHOULDER WIDTH	
RIGHT UPPER ARM	
LEFT UPPER ARM	
RIGHT FOREARM	
LEFT FOREARM	
WAIST	
HIPS	
RIGHT THIGH	
LEFT THIGH	
RIGHT CALF	
LEFT CALF	
BMI	
RMR	
RHR	

PART II

MAKE PROGRESS

Sustained weight loss is 95% diet. All diets work in the short term—any drastic change in eating habits will result in a radical change in your body. The key is finding foods you can live with in the long term. If the menu is too strict, you will cheat and slip back into old habits. Only you know your body and what will work for you.

The same goes for exercise. You have to find activities you like doing. If you don't, you will never exercise consistently. My knees are horrible, so I love DDP Yoga, swimming, and biking, all of which are easy on my knees. Find what works for you through trial and error. Try different approaches and paths. Weight loss is not a gentle, straight road. It is a curvy, frustrating, mountainous path with peaks and valleys.

Eat consistently, work out consistently, and journal consistently. Tweak, rinse, and repeat!

NOTES ON FILLING OUT THE JOURNAL PAGES

Now comes the fun part. Start with the day and date, then complete these logs as desired. At the very bottom, record the amount of sleep you got that night as well as how much water you drank that day. Keep in mind that your goal at the end of the next 90 days is to end up with as much information as possible.

Today's Activity: Mark your movement intention for the day: strength, cardio, or "other" if you are doing a combination of activities, or if you decide to take a rest day.

Muscle Group Focus: This section applies more to your strength days. What muscle groups are you trying to strengthen that day? Strength training is hard on the muscles. It is recommended to have rest days between lifting for specific muscle groups.

Strength: List each movement, the number of reps you accomplished, and the amount of weight lifted.

Cardio: List all of your cardio activities for the day: how far you biked, walked, ran, swam, how long your cardio activities lasted, and so on.

Macronutrients: Enter the total number of grams you consume of the listed macronutrients each day. The MyFitnessPal app is a great tool for calculating the macronutrients of your food. You can also use WebMD's Food Calculator (see Resources, page 115).

Evaluation: This star evaluation section is yours. Shade in the number of stars you feel is reflective of your day: five stars is a fantastic day, and one star is a terrible day. You decide the criteria on which to base your evaluation. It could be goal completion, diet compliance, how you feel about the day's weight loss progress, or a combination of these or any other factors. Mold these stars however you want.

DATE:_____ ❑ S ❑ M ❑ T ❑ W ❑ T ❑ F ❑ S

TODAY'S ACTIVITY:

❑ STRENGTH   ❑ CARDIO   ❑ OTHER _____

MUSCLE GROUP FOCUS:

❑ CHEST   ❑ ARMS   ❑ SHOULDERS   ❑ BACK   ❑ LEGS   ❑ CORE

STRENGTH						
EXERCISE	**SET 1**		**SET 2**		**SET 3**	
	Reps	Weight	Reps	Weight	Reps	Weight

CARDIO					
EXERCISE	Duration	km/mi	Speed	Incline	Calories

TOTAL LENGTH OF WORKOUT SESSION: _____MINUTES

MACRONUTRIENTS				
CARBS	**FATS**	**PROTEINS**	**SODIUM**	**SUGARS**

EVALUATION: ☆ ☆ ☆ ☆ ☆

SLEEP: _____HOURS   **WATER INTAKE:** _____oz/mL

DATE:_____ ❑ S ❑ M ❑ T ❑ W ❑ T ❑ F ❑ S

TODAY'S ACTIVITY:

❑ STRENGTH ❑ CARDIO ❑ OTHER _____

MUSCLE GROUP FOCUS:

❑ CHEST ❑ ARMS ❑ SHOULDERS ❑ BACK ❑ LEGS ❑ CORE

STRENGTH						
EXERCISE	**SET 1**		**SET 2**		**SET 3**	
	Reps	Weight	Reps	Weight	Reps	Weight

CARDIO					
EXERCISE	Duration	km/mi	Speed	Incline	Calories

TOTAL LENGTH OF WORKOUT SESSION: _____MINUTES

MACRONUTRIENTS				
CARBS	**FATS**	**PROTEINS**	**SODIUM**	**SUGARS**

EVALUATION: ☆ ☆ ☆ ☆ ☆

SLEEP: _____HOURS **WATER INTAKE:** _____oz/mL

DATE:_____   ❑ S ❑ M ❑ T ❑ W ❑ T ❑ F ❑ S

TODAY'S ACTIVITY:

❑ STRENGTH   ❑ CARDIO   ❑ OTHER _____

MUSCLE GROUP FOCUS:

❑ CHEST   ❑ ARMS   ❑ SHOULDERS   ❑ BACK   ❑ LEGS   ❑ CORE

STRENGTH						
EXERCISE	**SET 1**		**SET 2**		**SET 3**	
	Reps	Weight	Reps	Weight	Reps	Weight

CARDIO					
EXERCISE	Duration	km/mi	Speed	Incline	Calories

TOTAL LENGTH OF WORKOUT SESSION: _____MINUTES

MACRONUTRIENTS				
CARBS	**FATS**	**PROTEINS**	**SODIUM**	**SUGARS**

EVALUATION: ☆ ☆ ☆ ☆ ☆

SLEEP: _____HOURS   **WATER INTAKE:** _____oz/mL

DATE:_____ ❏ S ❏ M ❏ T ❏ W ❏ T ❏ F ❏ S

TODAY'S ACTIVITY:

❏ STRENGTH ❏ CARDIO ❏ OTHER _____

MUSCLE GROUP FOCUS:

❏ CHEST ❏ ARMS ❏ SHOULDERS ❏ BACK ❏ LEGS ❏ CORE

EXERCISE	SET 1		SET 2		SET 3	
	Reps	Weight	Reps	Weight	Reps	Weight

(STRENGTH table)

CARDIO					
EXERCISE	Duration	km/mi	Speed	Incline	Calories

TOTAL LENGTH OF WORKOUT SESSION: _____ MINUTES

MACRONUTRIENTS				
CARBS	FATS	PROTEINS	SODIUM	SUGARS

EVALUATION: ☆ ☆ ☆ ☆ ☆

SLEEP: _____ HOURS   **WATER INTAKE:** _____ oz/mL

DATE:_____ ❏ S ❏ M ❏ T ❏ W ❏ T ❏ F ❏ S

TODAY'S ACTIVITY:
❏ STRENGTH ❏ CARDIO ❏ OTHER _____

MUSCLE GROUP FOCUS:
❏ CHEST ❏ ARMS ❏ SHOULDERS ❏ BACK ❏ LEGS ❏ CORE

STRENGTH						
EXERCISE	**SET 1**		**SET 2**		**SET 3**	
	Reps	Weight	Reps	Weight	Reps	Weight

CARDIO					
EXERCISE	Duration	km/mi	Speed	Incline	Calories

TOTAL LENGTH OF WORKOUT SESSION: _____MINUTES

MACRONUTRIENTS				
CARBS	**FATS**	**PROTEINS**	**SODIUM**	**SUGARS**

EVALUATION: ☆ ☆ ☆ ☆ ☆

SLEEP: _____HOURS   **WATER INTAKE:** _____oz/mL

DATE:_____ ❑ S ❑ M ❑ T ❑ W ❑ T ❑ F ❑ S

TODAY'S ACTIVITY:

❑ STRENGTH ❑ CARDIO ❑ OTHER _____

MUSCLE GROUP FOCUS:

❑ CHEST ❑ ARMS ❑ SHOULDERS ❑ BACK ❑ LEGS ❑ CORE

STRENGTH						
EXERCISE	SET 1		SET 2		SET 3	
	Reps	Weight	Reps	Weight	Reps	Weight

CARDIO					
EXERCISE	Duration	km/mi	Speed	Incline	Calories

TOTAL LENGTH OF WORKOUT SESSION: _____MINUTES

MACRONUTRIENTS				
CARBS	FATS	PROTEINS	SODIUM	SUGARS

EVALUATION: ☆ ☆ ☆ ☆ ☆

SLEEP: _____HOURS   **WATER INTAKE:** _____oz/mL

DATE:_____   ❑ S ❑ M ❑ T ❑ W ❑ T ❑ F ❑ S

TODAY'S ACTIVITY:

❑ STRENGTH   ❑ CARDIO   ❑ OTHER _____

MUSCLE GROUP FOCUS:

❑ CHEST   ❑ ARMS   ❑ SHOULDERS   ❑ BACK   ❑ LEGS   ❑ CORE

STRENGTH						
EXERCISE	**SET 1**		**SET 2**		**SET 3**	
	Reps	Weight	Reps	Weight	Reps	Weight

CARDIO					
EXERCISE	Duration	km/mi	Speed	Incline	Calories

TOTAL LENGTH OF WORKOUT SESSION: _____MINUTES

MACRONUTRIENTS				
CARBS	**FATS**	**PROTEINS**	**SODIUM**	**SUGARS**

EVALUATION: ☆ ☆ ☆ ☆ ☆

SLEEP: _____HOURS   **WATER INTAKE:** _____oz/mL

DATE:_____ ❏ S ❏ M ❏ T ❏ W ❏ T ❏ F ❏ S

TODAY'S ACTIVITY:

❏ STRENGTH   ❏ CARDIO   ❏ OTHER _____

MUSCLE GROUP FOCUS:

❏ CHEST   ❏ ARMS   ❏ SHOULDERS   ❏ BACK   ❏ LEGS   ❏ CORE

STRENGTH						
EXERCISE	**SET 1**		**SET 2**		**SET 3**	
	Reps	Weight	Reps	Weight	Reps	Weight

CARDIO					
EXERCISE	Duration	km/mi	Speed	Incline	Calories

TOTAL LENGTH OF WORKOUT SESSION: _____MINUTES

MACRONUTRIENTS				
CARBS	**FATS**	**PROTEINS**	**SODIUM**	**SUGARS**

EVALUATION: ☆ ☆ ☆ ☆ ☆

SLEEP: _____HOURS   **WATER INTAKE:** _____oz/mL

DATE:_____ ❑ S ❑ M ❑ T ❑ W ❑ T ❑ F ❑ S

TODAY'S ACTIVITY:
❑ STRENGTH   ❑ CARDIO   ❑ OTHER _____

MUSCLE GROUP FOCUS:
❑ CHEST   ❑ ARMS   ❑ SHOULDERS   ❑ BACK   ❑ LEGS   ❑ CORE

STRENGTH						
EXERCISE	SET 1		SET 2		SET 3	
	Reps	Weight	Reps	Weight	Reps	Weight

CARDIO					
EXERCISE	Duration	km/mi	Speed	Incline	Calories

TOTAL LENGTH OF WORKOUT SESSION: _____ MINUTES

MACRONUTRIENTS				
CARBS	FATS	PROTEINS	SODIUM	SUGARS

EVALUATION: ☆ ☆ ☆ ☆ ☆

SLEEP: _____ HOURS   **WATER INTAKE:** _____ oz/mL

DATE:_____ ❑ S ❑ M ❑ T ❑ W ❑ T ❑ F ❑ S

TODAY'S ACTIVITY:

❑ STRENGTH   ❑ CARDIO   ❑ OTHER _____

MUSCLE GROUP FOCUS:

❑ CHEST   ❑ ARMS   ❑ SHOULDERS   ❑ BACK   ❑ LEGS   ❑ CORE

STRENGTH					
EXERCISE	**SET 1**		**SET 2**		**SET 3**	
	Reps	Weight	Reps	Weight	Reps	Weight

CARDIO					
EXERCISE	Duration	km/mi	Speed	Incline	Calories

TOTAL LENGTH OF WORKOUT SESSION: _____MINUTES

MACRONUTRIENTS				
CARBS	**FATS**	**PROTEINS**	**SODIUM**	**SUGARS**

EVALUATION: ☆ ☆ ☆ ☆ ☆

SLEEP: _____HOURS   **WATER INTAKE:** _____oz/mL

FITNESS MYTH #1:
As Long as You Exercise, Macronutrients Don't Matter

"You can't outwork a bad diet, bro!" I can't begin to count how many times I've heard Diamond Dallas Page say this over the years. It doesn't matter how hard you exercise: You can't outwork a bad diet. Weight loss begins and ends with the diet, period.

This journal allows you to easily track your intake of five key macronutrients: carbs, fats, proteins, sodium, and sugars. Diets exist in every combination of food groups, macronutrient percentages, eating time restrictions, proportion sizes, and eating methods, but inherent in any diet is the need to count the calories eaten. By tracking your macronutrient intake, you also track your caloric intake:

1 gram of protein = 4 calories

1 gram of carbohydrates = 4 calories

1 gram of fat = 9 calories

1 gram of sugar = 4 calories

1 gram of sodium = 0 calories

Breaking food down to the macronutrient level provides invaluable data on how your body processes it. In order to know whether a diet like a carnivore or a vegan is best for you, you need to know how much of the relevant macronutrients you consume when you perform at your peak.

I am insulin resistant. My body does not process most carbohydrates, sugar, or alcohol well. That means I operate best on a high-protein or low-carb diet. You have to track what you eat to know your body. Or, as Dallas also likes to say: "Listen to your body!"

DATE:_____ ❑ S ❑ M ❑ T ❑ W ❑ T ❑ F ❑ S

TODAY'S ACTIVITY:

❑ STRENGTH ❑ CARDIO ❑ OTHER _____

MUSCLE GROUP FOCUS:

❑ CHEST ❑ ARMS ❑ SHOULDERS ❑ BACK ❑ LEGS ❑ CORE

STRENGTH					
EXERCISE	**SET 1**		**SET 2**		**SET 3**	
	Reps	Weight	Reps	Weight	Reps	Weight

CARDIO					
EXERCISE	Duration	km/mi	Speed	Incline	Calories

TOTAL LENGTH OF WORKOUT SESSION: _____MINUTES

MACRONUTRIENTS				
CARBS	**FATS**	**PROTEINS**	**SODIUM**	**SUGARS**

EVALUATION: ☆ ☆ ☆ ☆ ☆

SLEEP: _____HOURS   **WATER INTAKE:** _____oz/mL

DATE:_____ ❑ S ❑ M ❑ T ❑ W ❑ T ❑ F ❑ S

TODAY'S ACTIVITY:
❑ STRENGTH ❑ CARDIO ❑ OTHER _____

MUSCLE GROUP FOCUS:
❑ CHEST ❑ ARMS ❑ SHOULDERS ❑ BACK ❑ LEGS ❑ CORE

EXERCISE	STRENGTH					
	SET 1		SET 2		SET 3	
	Reps	Weight	Reps	Weight	Reps	Weight

CARDIO					
EXERCISE	Duration	km/mi	Speed	Incline	Calories

TOTAL LENGTH OF WORKOUT SESSION: _____MINUTES

MACRONUTRIENTS				
CARBS	FATS	PROTEINS	SODIUM	SUGARS

EVALUATION: ☆ ☆ ☆ ☆ ☆

SLEEP: _____HOURS   **WATER INTAKE:** _____oz/mL

DATE:_____   ❏ S   ❏ M   ❏ T   ❏ W   ❏ T   ❏ F   ❏ S

TODAY'S ACTIVITY:

❏ STRENGTH   ❏ CARDIO   ❏ OTHER _____

MUSCLE GROUP FOCUS:

❏ CHEST   ❏ ARMS   ❏ SHOULDERS   ❏ BACK   ❏ LEGS   ❏ CORE

STRENGTH						
EXERCISE	**SET 1**		**SET 2**		**SET 3**	
	Reps	Weight	Reps	Weight	Reps	Weight

CARDIO					
EXERCISE	Duration	km/mi	Speed	Incline	Calories

TOTAL LENGTH OF WORKOUT SESSION: _____MINUTES

MACRONUTRIENTS				
CARBS	**FATS**	**PROTEINS**	**SODIUM**	**SUGARS**

EVALUATION: ☆ ☆ ☆ ☆ ☆

SLEEP: _____HOURS   **WATER INTAKE:** _____oz/mL

DATE:_____ ❏ S ❏ M ❏ T ❏ W ❏ T ❏ F ❏ S

TODAY'S ACTIVITY:

❏ STRENGTH   ❏ CARDIO   ❏ OTHER _____

MUSCLE GROUP FOCUS:

❏ CHEST   ❏ ARMS   ❏ SHOULDERS   ❏ BACK   ❏ LEGS   ❏ CORE

EXERCISE	STRENGTH					
	SET 1		SET 2		SET 3	
	Reps	Weight	Reps	Weight	Reps	Weight

CARDIO					
EXERCISE	Duration	km/mi	Speed	Incline	Calories

TOTAL LENGTH OF WORKOUT SESSION: _____MINUTES

MACRONUTRIENTS				
CARBS	FATS	PROTEINS	SODIUM	SUGARS

EVALUATION: ☆ ☆ ☆ ☆ ☆

SLEEP: _____HOURS   **WATER INTAKE:** _____oz/mL

DATE:_____ ❑ S ❑ M ❑ T ❑ W ❑ T ❑ F ❑ S

TODAY'S ACTIVITY:

❑ STRENGTH ❑ CARDIO ❑ OTHER _____

MUSCLE GROUP FOCUS:

❑ CHEST ❑ ARMS ❑ SHOULDERS ❑ BACK ❑ LEGS ❑ CORE

EXERCISE	SET 1		SET 2		SET 3	
	Reps	Weight	Reps	Weight	Reps	Weight

STRENGTH

EXERCISE	Duration	km/mi	Speed	Incline	Calories

CARDIO

TOTAL LENGTH OF WORKOUT SESSION: _____MINUTES

MACRONUTRIENTS				
CARBS	FATS	PROTEINS	SODIUM	SUGARS

EVALUATION: ☆ ☆ ☆ ☆ ☆

SLEEP: _____HOURS   **WATER INTAKE:** _____oz/mL

DATE:_____

❑ S ❑ M ❑ T ❑ W ❑ T ❑ F ❑ S

TODAY'S ACTIVITY:

❑ STRENGTH ❑ CARDIO ❑ OTHER _____

MUSCLE GROUP FOCUS:

❑ CHEST ❑ ARMS ❑ SHOULDERS ❑ BACK ❑ LEGS ❑ CORE

STRENGTH						
EXERCISE	SET 1		SET 2		SET 3	
	Reps	Weight	Reps	Weight	Reps	Weight

CARDIO					
EXERCISE	Duration	km/mi	Speed	Incline	Calories

TOTAL LENGTH OF WORKOUT SESSION: _____MINUTES

MACRONUTRIENTS				
CARBS	FATS	PROTEINS	SODIUM	SUGARS

EVALUATION: ☆ ☆ ☆ ☆ ☆

SLEEP: _____HOURS   **WATER INTAKE:** _____oz/mL

DATE:_____ ❏ S ❏ M ❏ T ❏ W ❏ T ❏ F ❏ S

TODAY'S ACTIVITY:

❏ STRENGTH   ❏ CARDIO   ❏ OTHER _____

MUSCLE GROUP FOCUS:

❏ CHEST   ❏ ARMS   ❏ SHOULDERS   ❏ BACK   ❏ LEGS   ❏ CORE

EXERCISE	SET 1		SET 2		SET 3	
	Reps	Weight	Reps	Weight	Reps	Weight

STRENGTH

CARDIO					
EXERCISE	Duration	km/mi	Speed	Incline	Calories

TOTAL LENGTH OF WORKOUT SESSION: _____MINUTES

MACRONUTRIENTS				
CARBS	FATS	PROTEINS	SODIUM	SUGARS

EVALUATION: ☆ ☆ ☆ ☆ ☆

SLEEP: _____HOURS   **WATER INTAKE:** _____oz/mL

DATE:_____ ❑ S ❑ M ❑ T ❑ W ❑ T ❑ F ❑ S

TODAY'S ACTIVITY:
❑ STRENGTH ❑ CARDIO ❑ OTHER _____

MUSCLE GROUP FOCUS:
❑ CHEST ❑ ARMS ❑ SHOULDERS ❑ BACK ❑ LEGS ❑ CORE

STRENGTH						
EXERCISE	**SET 1**		**SET 2**		**SET 3**	
	Reps	Weight	Reps	Weight	Reps	Weight

CARDIO					
EXERCISE	Duration	km/mi	Speed	Incline	Calories

TOTAL LENGTH OF WORKOUT SESSION: _____ MINUTES

MACRONUTRIENTS				
CARBS	**FATS**	**PROTEINS**	**SODIUM**	**SUGARS**

EVALUATION: ☆ ☆ ☆ ☆ ☆

SLEEP: _____ HOURS   **WATER INTAKE:** _____ oz/mL

DATE:_____   ❑ S ❑ M ❑ T ❑ W ❑ T ❑ F ❑ S

TODAY'S ACTIVITY:

❑ STRENGTH   ❑ CARDIO   ❑ OTHER _____

MUSCLE GROUP FOCUS:

❑ CHEST   ❑ ARMS   ❑ SHOULDERS   ❑ BACK   ❑ LEGS   ❑ CORE

STRENGTH						
EXERCISE	**SET 1**		**SET 2**		**SET 3**	
	Reps	Weight	Reps	Weight	Reps	Weight

CARDIO					
EXERCISE	Duration	km/mi	Speed	Incline	Calories

TOTAL LENGTH OF WORKOUT SESSION: _____ MINUTES

MACRONUTRIENTS				
CARBS	**FATS**	**PROTEINS**	**SODIUM**	**SUGARS**

EVALUATION: ☆ ☆ ☆ ☆ ☆

SLEEP: _____ HOURS   **WATER INTAKE:** _____ oz/mL

DATE:_____ ❑ S ❑ M ❑ T ❑ W ❑ T ❑ F ❑ S

TODAY'S ACTIVITY:

❑ STRENGTH ❑ CARDIO ❑ OTHER _____

MUSCLE GROUP FOCUS:

❑ CHEST ❑ ARMS ❑ SHOULDERS ❑ BACK ❑ LEGS ❑ CORE

STRENGTH						
EXERCISE	**SET 1**		**SET 2**		**SET 3**	
	Reps	Weight	Reps	Weight	Reps	Weight

CARDIO					
EXERCISE	Duration	km/mi	Speed	Incline	Calories

TOTAL LENGTH OF WORKOUT SESSION: _____MINUTES

MACRONUTRIENTS				
CARBS	**FATS**	**PROTEINS**	**SODIUM**	**SUGARS**

EVALUATION: ☆ ☆ ☆ ☆ ☆

SLEEP: _____HOURS **WATER INTAKE:** _____oz/mL

FITNESS MYTH #2:
You Have to Lead with Cardio

Your body needs a certain number of calories to perform the basic functions of life. This daily essential caloric requirement is your basal metabolic rate (BMR) or resting metabolic rate (RMR). These terms are not identical but very similar. For our purposes, I will refer to your RMR. Any extra activity beyond your RMR will cause you to burn calories. And if the amount of calories burned by this extra activity plus your RMR is greater than your caloric intake, you will lose weight. It is just that simple.

A great dieting calculator like the Flexible Dieting Macro Calculator from the *Healthy Eater* blog (see Resources, page 115) can provide you with an estimate of the daily caloric intake you need to maintain your current weight, lose weight, or lose weight quickly. You can use one of these numbers as your expected daily caloric intake goal.

Cardio is simply one method of burning extra calories past your RMR. There are many other ways to burn calories, including practically any activity you might do outside of your normal routine: weight lifting, yoga, jujitsu, biking, walking, Pilates, spin class, rowing, yard work, swimming, rugby, soccer, badminton, jumping rope, table tennis, bird-watching, fishing, gardening, hiking, boxing—the list goes on and on. Why choose a method you don't like? Find a pursuit that is enjoyable to you. If you don't like the activity, don't do it. Get to experimenting!

MEASUREMENT LOG 1

DATE:_____

NECK	
CHEST	
SHOULDER WIDTH	
RIGHT UPPER ARM	
LEFT UPPER ARM	
RIGHT FOREARM	
LEFT FOREARM	
WAIST	
HIPS	
RIGHT THIGH	
LEFT THIGH	
RIGHT CALF	
LEFT CALF	
BMI	
RMR	
RHR	

DATE:_____ ❏ S ❏ M ❏ T ❏ W ❏ T ❏ F ❏ S

TODAY'S ACTIVITY:

❏ STRENGTH ❏ CARDIO ❏ OTHER _____

MUSCLE GROUP FOCUS:

❏ CHEST ❏ ARMS ❏ SHOULDERS ❏ BACK ❏ LEGS ❏ CORE

STRENGTH						
EXERCISE	**SET 1**		**SET 2**		**SET 3**	
	Reps	Weight	Reps	Weight	Reps	Weight

CARDIO					
EXERCISE	Duration	km/mi	Speed	Incline	Calories

TOTAL LENGTH OF WORKOUT SESSION: _____MINUTES

MACRONUTRIENTS				
CARBS	**FATS**	**PROTEINS**	**SODIUM**	**SUGARS**

EVALUATION: ☆ ☆ ☆ ☆ ☆

SLEEP: _____HOURS **WATER INTAKE:** _____oz/mL

DATE:_____   ❏ S ❏ M ❏ T ❏ W ❏ T ❏ F ❏ S

TODAY'S ACTIVITY:

❏ STRENGTH   ❏ CARDIO   ❏ OTHER _____

MUSCLE GROUP FOCUS:

❏ CHEST   ❏ ARMS   ❏ SHOULDERS   ❏ BACK   ❏ LEGS   ❏ CORE

STRENGTH						
EXERCISE	**SET 1**		**SET 2**		**SET 3**	
	Reps	Weight	Reps	Weight	Reps	Weight

CARDIO					
EXERCISE	Duration	km/mi	Speed	Incline	Calories

TOTAL LENGTH OF WORKOUT SESSION: _____MINUTES

MACRONUTRIENTS				
CARBS	**FATS**	**PROTEINS**	**SODIUM**	**SUGARS**

EVALUATION: ☆ ☆ ☆ ☆ ☆

SLEEP: _____HOURS   **WATER INTAKE:** _____oz/mL

DATE:_____ ❏ S ❏ M ❏ T ❏ W ❏ T ❏ F ❏ S

TODAY'S ACTIVITY:

❏ STRENGTH   ❏ CARDIO   ❏ OTHER _____

MUSCLE GROUP FOCUS:

❏ CHEST   ❏ ARMS   ❏ SHOULDERS   ❏ BACK   ❏ LEGS   ❏ CORE

STRENGTH						
EXERCISE	**SET 1**		**SET 2**		**SET 3**	
	Reps	Weight	Reps	Weight	Reps	Weight

CARDIO					
EXERCISE	Duration	km/mi	Speed	Incline	Calories

TOTAL LENGTH OF WORKOUT SESSION: _____MINUTES

MACRONUTRIENTS				
CARBS	**FATS**	**PROTEINS**	**SODIUM**	**SUGARS**

EVALUATION: ☆ ☆ ☆ ☆ ☆

SLEEP: _____HOURS   **WATER INTAKE:** _____oz/mL

DATE:_____ ❑ S ❑ M ❑ T ❑ W ❑ T ❑ F ❑ S

TODAY'S ACTIVITY:

❑ STRENGTH ❑ CARDIO ❑ OTHER _____

MUSCLE GROUP FOCUS:

❑ CHEST ❑ ARMS ❑ SHOULDERS ❑ BACK ❑ LEGS ❑ CORE

EXERCISE	SET 1		SET 2		SET 3	
	Reps	Weight	Reps	Weight	Reps	Weight

STRENGTH

CARDIO					
EXERCISE	Duration	km/mi	Speed	Incline	Calories

TOTAL LENGTH OF WORKOUT SESSION: _____MINUTES

MACRONUTRIENTS				
CARBS	FATS	PROTEINS	SODIUM	SUGARS

EVALUATION: ☆ ☆ ☆ ☆ ☆

SLEEP: _____HOURS   **WATER INTAKE:** _____oz/mL

DATE:_____ ❑ S ❑ M ❑ T ❑ W ❑ T ❑ F ❑ S

TODAY'S ACTIVITY:

❑ STRENGTH   ❑ CARDIO   ❑ OTHER _____

MUSCLE GROUP FOCUS:

❑ CHEST   ❑ ARMS   ❑ SHOULDERS   ❑ BACK   ❑ LEGS   ❑ CORE

STRENGTH						
EXERCISE	SET 1		SET 2		SET 3	
	Reps	Weight	Reps	Weight	Reps	Weight

CARDIO					
EXERCISE	Duration	km/mi	Speed	Incline	Calories

TOTAL LENGTH OF WORKOUT SESSION: _____ MINUTES

MACRONUTRIENTS				
CARBS	FATS	PROTEINS	SODIUM	SUGARS

EVALUATION: ☆ ☆ ☆ ☆ ☆

SLEEP: _____ HOURS   **WATER INTAKE:** _____ oz/mL

DATE:_____ ❑ S ❑ M ❑ T ❑ W ❑ T ❑ F ❑ S

TODAY'S ACTIVITY:

❑ STRENGTH ❑ CARDIO ❑ OTHER _____

MUSCLE GROUP FOCUS:

❑ CHEST ❑ ARMS ❑ SHOULDERS ❑ BACK ❑ LEGS ❑ CORE

STRENGTH						
EXERCISE	**SET 1**		**SET 2**		**SET 3**	
	Reps	Weight	Reps	Weight	Reps	Weight

CARDIO					
EXERCISE	Duration	km/mi	Speed	Incline	Calories

TOTAL LENGTH OF WORKOUT SESSION: _____MINUTES

MACRONUTRIENTS				
CARBS	**FATS**	**PROTEINS**	**SODIUM**	**SUGARS**

EVALUATION: ☆ ☆ ☆ ☆ ☆

SLEEP: _____HOURS **WATER INTAKE:** _____oz/mL

DATE:_____ ❑ S ❑ M ❑ T ❑ W ❑ T ❑ F ❑ S

TODAY'S ACTIVITY:

❑ STRENGTH ❑ CARDIO ❑ OTHER _____

MUSCLE GROUP FOCUS:

❑ CHEST ❑ ARMS ❑ SHOULDERS ❑ BACK ❑ LEGS ❑ CORE

EXERCISE	SET 1		SET 2		SET 3	
	Reps	Weight	Reps	Weight	Reps	Weight

STRENGTH

EXERCISE	Duration	km/mi	Speed	Incline	Calories

CARDIO

TOTAL LENGTH OF WORKOUT SESSION: _____ MINUTES

CARBS	FATS	PROTEINS	SODIUM	SUGARS

MACRONUTRIENTS

EVALUATION: ☆ ☆ ☆ ☆ ☆

SLEEP: _____ HOURS **WATER INTAKE:** _____ oz/mL

DATE:_____   ❑ S ❑ M ❑ T ❑ W ❑ T ❑ F ❑ S

TODAY'S ACTIVITY:

❑ STRENGTH   ❑ CARDIO   ❑ OTHER _____

MUSCLE GROUP FOCUS:

❑ CHEST   ❑ ARMS   ❑ SHOULDERS   ❑ BACK   ❑ LEGS   ❑ CORE

STRENGTH						
EXERCISE	SET 1		SET 2		SET 3	
	Reps	Weight	Reps	Weight	Reps	Weight

CARDIO					
EXERCISE	Duration	km/mi	Speed	Incline	Calories

TOTAL LENGTH OF WORKOUT SESSION: _____MINUTES

MACRONUTRIENTS				
CARBS	FATS	PROTEINS	SODIUM	SUGARS

EVALUATION: ☆ ☆ ☆ ☆ ☆

SLEEP: _____HOURS   **WATER INTAKE:** _____oz/mL

DATE:_____   ❑ S ❑ M ❑ T ❑ W ❑ T ❑ F ❑ S

TODAY'S ACTIVITY:

❑ STRENGTH   ❑ CARDIO   ❑ OTHER _____

MUSCLE GROUP FOCUS:

❑ CHEST   ❑ ARMS   ❑ SHOULDERS   ❑ BACK   ❑ LEGS   ❑ CORE

STRENGTH						
EXERCISE	SET 1		SET 2		SET 3	
	Reps	Weight	Reps	Weight	Reps	Weight

CARDIO					
EXERCISE	Duration	km/mi	Speed	Incline	Calories

TOTAL LENGTH OF WORKOUT SESSION: _____MINUTES

MACRONUTRIENTS				
CARBS	FATS	PROTEINS	SODIUM	SUGARS

EVALUATION: ☆ ☆ ☆ ☆ ☆

SLEEP: _____HOURS   **WATER INTAKE:** _____oz/mL

DATE:_____   ❏ S ❏ M ❏ T ❏ W ❏ T ❏ F ❏ S

TODAY'S ACTIVITY:
❏ STRENGTH   ❏ CARDIO   ❏ OTHER _____

MUSCLE GROUP FOCUS:
❏ CHEST   ❏ ARMS   ❏ SHOULDERS   ❏ BACK   ❏ LEGS   ❏ CORE

STRENGTH						
EXERCISE	**SET 1**		**SET 2**		**SET 3**	
	Reps	Weight	Reps	Weight	Reps	Weight

CARDIO					
EXERCISE	Duration	km/mi	Speed	Incline	Calories

TOTAL LENGTH OF WORKOUT SESSION: _____MINUTES

MACRONUTRIENTS				
CARBS	**FATS**	**PROTEINS**	**SODIUM**	**SUGARS**

EVALUATION: ☆ ☆ ☆ ☆ ☆

SLEEP: _____HOURS   **WATER INTAKE:** _____oz/mL

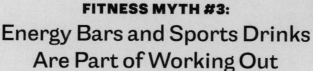

FITNESS MYTH #3:

Energy Bars and Sports Drinks Are Part of Working Out

Diamond Dallas Page made me watch three movies as part of my fitness journey: *The Resurrection of Jake the Snake*; *Food, Inc.*; and *Genetic Roulette: The Gamble of Our Lives*. Two of these movies are about the food we put in our mouths, and the basic premise of these movies is that processed food is trash.

Modern agribusiness has changed the nature of our food. We leave its processing to profit-driven companies that add artificial ingredients, genetically modify it beyond recognition, and then wrap it up in a convenient package for us to eat. These processed foods are available in every corner store and grocery store, and their convenience and low cost make them dangerous.

I know not all processed food is terrible. As a general rule, though, you should try to eat food in its most natural form. The more processed the food, the more you should stay away from it. I try to eat organically grown, non-GMO, and grass-fed products. Our bodies have been digesting this type of food for hundreds of thousands of years, and they're built to thrive on it.

I think energy bars and sports drinks are like fishing lures. Some lures are designed to catch a fish, and others are designed to catch a fisher. Most of the food substitutes and supplements on the market are designed only to catch consumers, not to actually improve your health. My personal preference is not to grab the protein bar or shake but instead to eat naturally. That is just my opinion; take it or leave it as you will.

DATE:_____   ❑ S ❑ M ❑ T ❑ W ❑ T ❑ F ❑ S

TODAY'S ACTIVITY:
❑ STRENGTH   ❑ CARDIO   ❑ OTHER _____

MUSCLE GROUP FOCUS:
❑ CHEST   ❑ ARMS   ❑ SHOULDERS   ❑ BACK   ❑ LEGS   ❑ CORE

STRENGTH						
EXERCISE	SET 1		SET 2		SET 3	
	Reps	Weight	Reps	Weight	Reps	Weight

CARDIO					
EXERCISE	Duration	km/mi	Speed	Incline	Calories

TOTAL LENGTH OF WORKOUT SESSION: _____MINUTES

MACRONUTRIENTS				
CARBS	FATS	PROTEINS	SODIUM	SUGARS

EVALUATION: ☆ ☆ ☆ ☆ ☆

SLEEP: _____HOURS   **WATER INTAKE:** _____oz/mL

DATE:_____ ❏ S ❏ M ❏ T ❏ W ❏ T ❏ F ❏ S

TODAY'S ACTIVITY:

❏ STRENGTH   ❏ CARDIO   ❏ OTHER _____

MUSCLE GROUP FOCUS:

❏ CHEST   ❏ ARMS   ❏ SHOULDERS   ❏ BACK   ❏ LEGS   ❏ CORE

STRENGTH						
EXERCISE	SET 1		SET 2		SET 3	
	Reps	Weight	Reps	Weight	Reps	Weight

CARDIO					
EXERCISE	Duration	km/mi	Speed	Incline	Calories

TOTAL LENGTH OF WORKOUT SESSION: _____MINUTES

MACRONUTRIENTS				
CARBS	FATS	PROTEINS	SODIUM	SUGARS

EVALUATION: ☆ ☆ ☆ ☆ ☆

SLEEP: _____HOURS   **WATER INTAKE:** _____oz/mL

DATE:_____   ❏ S   ❏ M   ❏ T   ❏ W   ❏ T   ❏ F   ❏ S

TODAY'S ACTIVITY:

❏ STRENGTH   ❏ CARDIO   ❏ OTHER _____

MUSCLE GROUP FOCUS:

❏ CHEST   ❏ ARMS   ❏ SHOULDERS   ❏ BACK   ❏ LEGS   ❏ CORE

STRENGTH						
EXERCISE	**SET 1**		**SET 2**		**SET 3**	
	Reps	Weight	Reps	Weight	Reps	Weight

CARDIO					
EXERCISE	Duration	km/mi	Speed	Incline	Calories

TOTAL LENGTH OF WORKOUT SESSION: _____MINUTES

MACRONUTRIENTS				
CARBS	**FATS**	**PROTEINS**	**SODIUM**	**SUGARS**

EVALUATION: ☆ ☆ ☆ ☆ ☆

SLEEP: _____HOURS   **WATER INTAKE:** _____oz/mL

DATE:_____ ❑ S ❑ M ❑ T ❑ W ❑ T ❑ F ❑ S

TODAY'S ACTIVITY:

❑ STRENGTH ❑ CARDIO ❑ OTHER _____

MUSCLE GROUP FOCUS:

❑ CHEST ❑ ARMS ❑ SHOULDERS ❑ BACK ❑ LEGS ❑ CORE

STRENGTH						
EXERCISE	**SET 1**		**SET 2**		**SET 3**	
	Reps	Weight	Reps	Weight	Reps	Weight

CARDIO					
EXERCISE	Duration	km/mi	Speed	Incline	Calories

TOTAL LENGTH OF WORKOUT SESSION: _____MINUTES

MACRONUTRIENTS				
CARBS	**FATS**	**PROTEINS**	**SODIUM**	**SUGARS**

EVALUATION: ☆ ☆ ☆ ☆ ☆

SLEEP: _____HOURS   **WATER INTAKE:** _____oz/mL

DATE:_____ ❏ S ❏ M ❏ T ❏ W ❏ T ❏ F ❏ S

TODAY'S ACTIVITY:

❏ STRENGTH ❏ CARDIO ❏ OTHER _____

MUSCLE GROUP FOCUS:

❏ CHEST ❏ ARMS ❏ SHOULDERS ❏ BACK ❏ LEGS ❏ CORE

EXERCISE	SET 1		SET 2		SET 3	
	Reps	Weight	Reps	Weight	Reps	Weight

STRENGTH

EXERCISE	Duration	km/mi	Speed	Incline	Calories

CARDIO

TOTAL LENGTH OF WORKOUT SESSION: _____MINUTES

CARBS	FATS	PROTEINS	SODIUM	SUGARS

MACRONUTRIENTS

EVALUATION: ☆ ☆ ☆ ☆ ☆

SLEEP: _____HOURS **WATER INTAKE:** _____oz/mL

DATE:_____   ❑ S ❑ M ❑ T ❑ W ❑ T ❑ F ❑ S

TODAY'S ACTIVITY:

❑ STRENGTH   ❑ CARDIO   ❑ OTHER_____

MUSCLE GROUP FOCUS:

❑ CHEST   ❑ ARMS   ❑ SHOULDERS   ❑ BACK   ❑ LEGS   ❑ CORE

	STRENGTH					
EXERCISE	SET 1		SET 2		SET 3	
	Reps	Weight	Reps	Weight	Reps	Weight

CARDIO					
EXERCISE	Duration	km/mi	Speed	Incline	Calories

TOTAL LENGTH OF WORKOUT SESSION: _____MINUTES

MACRONUTRIENTS				
CARBS	**FATS**	**PROTEINS**	**SODIUM**	**SUGARS**

EVALUATION: ☆ ☆ ☆ ☆ ☆

SLEEP: _____HOURS   **WATER INTAKE:** _____oz/mL

DATE:_____ ❑ S ❑ M ❑ T ❑ W ❑ T ❑ F ❑ S

TODAY'S ACTIVITY:

❑ STRENGTH   ❑ CARDIO   ❑ OTHER _____

MUSCLE GROUP FOCUS:

❑ CHEST   ❑ ARMS   ❑ SHOULDERS   ❑ BACK   ❑ LEGS   ❑ CORE

STRENGTH						
EXERCISE	SET 1		SET 2		SET 3	
	Reps	Weight	Reps	Weight	Reps	Weight

CARDIO					
EXERCISE	Duration	km/mi	Speed	Incline	Calories

TOTAL LENGTH OF WORKOUT SESSION: _____MINUTES

MACRONUTRIENTS				
CARBS	FATS	PROTEINS	SODIUM	SUGARS

EVALUATION: ☆ ☆ ☆ ☆ ☆

SLEEP: _____HOURS   **WATER INTAKE:** _____oz/mL

DATE:_____   ❏ S   ❏ M   ❏ T   ❏ W   ❏ T   ❏ F   ❏ S

TODAY'S ACTIVITY:

❏ STRENGTH   ❏ CARDIO   ❏ OTHER _____

MUSCLE GROUP FOCUS:

❏ CHEST   ❏ ARMS   ❏ SHOULDERS   ❏ BACK   ❏ LEGS   ❏ CORE

STRENGTH						
EXERCISE	SET 1		SET 2		SET 3	
	Reps	Weight	Reps	Weight	Reps	Weight

CARDIO					
EXERCISE	Duration	km/mi	Speed	Incline	Calories

TOTAL LENGTH OF WORKOUT SESSION: _____MINUTES

MACRONUTRIENTS				
CARBS	FATS	PROTEINS	SODIUM	SUGARS

EVALUATION: ☆ ☆ ☆ ☆ ☆

SLEEP: _____HOURS   **WATER INTAKE:** _____oz/mL

DATE:_____   ❏ S ❏ M ❏ T ❏ W ❏ T ❏ F ❏ S

TODAY'S ACTIVITY:

❏ STRENGTH   ❏ CARDIO   ❏ OTHER _____

MUSCLE GROUP FOCUS:

❏ CHEST   ❏ ARMS   ❏ SHOULDERS   ❏ BACK   ❏ LEGS   ❏ CORE

STRENGTH						
EXERCISE	**SET 1**		**SET 2**		**SET 3**	
	Reps	Weight	Reps	Weight	Reps	Weight

CARDIO					
EXERCISE	Duration	km/mi	Speed	Incline	Calories

TOTAL LENGTH OF WORKOUT SESSION: _____MINUTES

MACRONUTRIENTS				
CARBS	**FATS**	**PROTEINS**	**SODIUM**	**SUGARS**

EVALUATION: ☆ ☆ ☆ ☆ ☆

SLEEP: _____HOURS   **WATER INTAKE:** _____oz/mL

DATE:_____ ❑ S ❑ M ❑ T ❑ W ❑ T ❑ F ❑ S

TODAY'S ACTIVITY:

❑ STRENGTH   ❑ CARDIO   ❑ OTHER _____

MUSCLE GROUP FOCUS:

❑ CHEST   ❑ ARMS   ❑ SHOULDERS   ❑ BACK   ❑ LEGS   ❑ CORE

STRENGTH						
EXERCISE	**SET 1**		**SET 2**		**SET 3**	
	Reps	Weight	Reps	Weight	Reps	Weight

CARDIO					
EXERCISE	Duration	km/mi	Speed	Incline	Calories

TOTAL LENGTH OF WORKOUT SESSION: _____MINUTES

MACRONUTRIENTS				
CARBS	**FATS**	**PROTEINS**	**SODIUM**	**SUGARS**

EVALUATION: ☆ ☆ ☆ ☆ ☆

SLEEP: _____HOURS   **WATER INTAKE:** _____oz/mL

FITNESS MYTH #4:
Low-Fat Foods Are Essential to Every Diet

My whole life, I have been told that I need to eat a low-fat diet to stay healthy. Since the 1980s, the low-fat diet has loomed large over American culture. Every doctor that has treated me has opined the benefits of a low-fat lifestyle. But low-fat has never worked for me.

In a 2008 article published in the *Journal of the History of Medicine and Allied Science*, medical historian Ann F. La Berge traced the history of the low-fat diet and detailed this dogma's dominance of American culture. It is an excellent article; I highly encourage you to read it (see References, page 116).

La Berge noted that, thankfully, attitudes toward total fat consumption became less extreme in the 2000s: the USDA Dietary Guidelines issued in January 2005 increased the top recommended percentage of fat an individual should consume from 30 percent to 35 percent, with a suggested range of 20 percent to 35 percent. The focus shifted to reducing the consumption of processed foods, which contain unhealthy fats alongside high sugar and salt content.

I believe this was a positive move toward diets that are more natural for most people. You should try to eat good fats, such as avocados, walnuts, vegetable oils, and fatty fish. But the most important thing is to tweak your diet to fit your body. There is no one size that fits all. Eat what works for you.

MEASUREMENT LOG 2

DATE:_____

NECK			
CHEST			
SHOULDER WIDTH			
RIGHT UPPER ARM			
LEFT UPPER ARM			
RIGHT FOREARM			
LEFT FOREARM			
WAIST			
HIPS			
RIGHT THIGH			
LEFT THIGH			
RIGHT CALF			
LEFT CALF			
BMI			
RMR			
RHR			

DATE:_____   ❏ S ❏ M ❏ T ❏ W ❏ T ❏ F ❏ S

TODAY'S ACTIVITY:
❏ STRENGTH   ❏ CARDIO   ❏ OTHER _____

MUSCLE GROUP FOCUS:
❏ CHEST   ❏ ARMS   ❏ SHOULDERS   ❏ BACK   ❏ LEGS   ❏ CORE

EXERCISE	STRENGTH					
	SET 1		SET 2		SET 3	
	Reps	Weight	Reps	Weight	Reps	Weight

CARDIO					
EXERCISE	Duration	km/mi	Speed	Incline	Calories

TOTAL LENGTH OF WORKOUT SESSION: _____MINUTES

MACRONUTRIENTS				
CARBS	FATS	PROTEINS	SODIUM	SUGARS

EVALUATION: ☆ ☆ ☆ ☆ ☆

SLEEP: _____HOURS   **WATER INTAKE:** _____oz/mL

DATE:_____ ❑ S ❑ M ❑ T ❑ W ❑ T ❑ F ❑ S

TODAY'S ACTIVITY:

❑ STRENGTH ❑ CARDIO ❑ OTHER_____

MUSCLE GROUP FOCUS:

❑ CHEST ❑ ARMS ❑ SHOULDERS ❑ BACK ❑ LEGS ❑ CORE

EXERCISE	STRENGTH					
	SET 1		SET 2		SET 3	
	Reps	Weight	Reps	Weight	Reps	Weight

CARDIO					
EXERCISE	Duration	km/mi	Speed	Incline	Calories

TOTAL LENGTH OF WORKOUT SESSION: _____MINUTES

MACRONUTRIENTS				
CARBS	FATS	PROTEINS	SODIUM	SUGARS

EVALUATION: ☆ ☆ ☆ ☆ ☆

SLEEP: _____HOURS **WATER INTAKE:** _____oz/mL

DATE:_____   ❑ S ❑ M ❑ T ❑ W ❑ T ❑ F ❑ S

TODAY'S ACTIVITY:
❑ STRENGTH   ❑ CARDIO   ❑ OTHER _____

MUSCLE GROUP FOCUS:
❑ CHEST   ❑ ARMS   ❑ SHOULDERS   ❑ BACK   ❑ LEGS   ❑ CORE

STRENGTH						
EXERCISE	**SET 1**		**SET 2**		**SET 3**	
	Reps	Weight	Reps	Weight	Reps	Weight

CARDIO					
EXERCISE	Duration	km/mi	Speed	Incline	Calories

TOTAL LENGTH OF WORKOUT SESSION: _____MINUTES

MACRONUTRIENTS				
CARBS	**FATS**	**PROTEINS**	**SODIUM**	**SUGARS**

EVALUATION: ☆ ☆ ☆ ☆ ☆

SLEEP:_____HOURS   **WATER INTAKE:**_____oz/mL

DATE:_____ ❑ S ❑ M ❑ T ❑ W ❑ T ❑ F ❑ S

TODAY'S ACTIVITY:

❑ STRENGTH   ❑ CARDIO   ❑ OTHER _____

MUSCLE GROUP FOCUS:

❑ CHEST   ❑ ARMS   ❑ SHOULDERS   ❑ BACK   ❑ LEGS   ❑ CORE

STRENGTH						
EXERCISE	SET 1		SET 2		SET 3	
	Reps	Weight	Reps	Weight	Reps	Weight

CARDIO					
EXERCISE	Duration	km/mi	Speed	Incline	Calories

TOTAL LENGTH OF WORKOUT SESSION: _____MINUTES

MACRONUTRIENTS				
CARBS	FATS	PROTEINS	SODIUM	SUGARS

EVALUATION: ☆ ☆ ☆ ☆ ☆

SLEEP: _____HOURS   **WATER INTAKE:** _____oz/mL

DATE:_____ ❑ S ❑ M ❑ T ❑ W ❑ T ❑ F ❑ S

TODAY'S ACTIVITY:

❑ STRENGTH   ❑ CARDIO   ❑ OTHER _____

MUSCLE GROUP FOCUS:

❑ CHEST   ❑ ARMS   ❑ SHOULDERS   ❑ BACK   ❑ LEGS   ❑ CORE

EXERCISE	SET 1		SET 2		SET 3	
	Reps	Weight	Reps	Weight	Reps	Weight

STRENGTH

EXERCISE	Duration	km/mi	Speed	Incline	Calories

CARDIO

TOTAL LENGTH OF WORKOUT SESSION: _____MINUTES

CARBS	FATS	PROTEINS	SODIUM	SUGARS

MACRONUTRIENTS

EVALUATION: ☆ ☆ ☆ ☆ ☆

SLEEP: _____HOURS   **WATER INTAKE:** _____oz/mL

DATE:_____   ❑ S   ❑ M   ❑ T   ❑ W   ❑ T   ❑ F   ❑ S

TODAY'S ACTIVITY:

❑ STRENGTH   ❑ CARDIO   ❑ OTHER _____

MUSCLE GROUP FOCUS:

❑ CHEST   ❑ ARMS   ❑ SHOULDERS   ❑ BACK   ❑ LEGS   ❑ CORE

	STRENGTH						
EXERCISE	**SET 1**		**SET 2**		**SET 3**		
	Reps	Weight	Reps	Weight	Reps	Weight	

CARDIO					
EXERCISE	Duration	km/mi	Speed	Incline	Calories

TOTAL LENGTH OF WORKOUT SESSION: _____MINUTES

MACRONUTRIENTS				
CARBS	**FATS**	**PROTEINS**	**SODIUM**	**SUGARS**

EVALUATION: ☆ ☆ ☆ ☆ ☆

SLEEP: _____HOURS   **WATER INTAKE:** _____oz/mL

DATE:_____ ❑ S ❑ M ❑ T ❑ W ❑ T ❑ F ❑ S

TODAY'S ACTIVITY:

❑ STRENGTH   ❑ CARDIO   ❑ OTHER _____

MUSCLE GROUP FOCUS:

❑ CHEST   ❑ ARMS   ❑ SHOULDERS   ❑ BACK   ❑ LEGS   ❑ CORE

EXERCISE	STRENGTH					
	SET 1		SET 2		SET 3	
	Reps	Weight	Reps	Weight	Reps	Weight

CARDIO					
EXERCISE	Duration	km/mi	Speed	Incline	Calories

TOTAL LENGTH OF WORKOUT SESSION: _____ MINUTES

MACRONUTRIENTS				
CARBS	FATS	PROTEINS	SODIUM	SUGARS

EVALUATION: ☆ ☆ ☆ ☆ ☆

SLEEP: _____ HOURS   **WATER INTAKE:** _____ oz/mL

DATE:_____   ❏ S ❏ M ❏ T ❏ W ❏ T ❏ F ❏ S

TODAY'S ACTIVITY:

❏ STRENGTH   ❏ CARDIO   ❏ OTHER _____

MUSCLE GROUP FOCUS:

❏ CHEST   ❏ ARMS   ❏ SHOULDERS   ❏ BACK   ❏ LEGS   ❏ CORE

	STRENGTH							
EXERCISE	**SET 1**		**SET 2**			**SET 3**		
	Reps	Weight	Reps	Weight		Reps	Weight	

CARDIO					
EXERCISE	Duration	km/mi	Speed	Incline	Calories

TOTAL LENGTH OF WORKOUT SESSION: _____MINUTES

MACRONUTRIENTS				
CARBS	**FATS**	**PROTEINS**	**SODIUM**	**SUGARS**

EVALUATION: ☆ ☆ ☆ ☆ ☆

SLEEP: _____HOURS   **WATER INTAKE:** _____oz/mL

DATE:_____   ❑ S ❑ M ❑ T ❑ W ❑ T ❑ F ❑ S

TODAY'S ACTIVITY:

❑ STRENGTH   ❑ CARDIO   ❑ OTHER _____

MUSCLE GROUP FOCUS:

❑ CHEST   ❑ ARMS   ❑ SHOULDERS   ❑ BACK   ❑ LEGS   ❑ CORE

STRENGTH						
EXERCISE	**SET 1**		**SET 2**		**SET 3**	
	Reps	Weight	Reps	Weight	Reps	Weight

CARDIO					
EXERCISE	Duration	km/mi	Speed	Incline	Calories

TOTAL LENGTH OF WORKOUT SESSION: _____MINUTES

MACRONUTRIENTS				
CARBS	**FATS**	**PROTEINS**	**SODIUM**	**SUGARS**

EVALUATION: ☆ ☆ ☆ ☆ ☆

SLEEP: _____HOURS   **WATER INTAKE:** _____oz/mL

DATE:_____ ❏ S ❏ M ❏ T ❏ W ❏ T ❏ F ❏ S

TODAY'S ACTIVITY:

❏ STRENGTH ❏ CARDIO ❏ OTHER _____

MUSCLE GROUP FOCUS:

❏ CHEST ❏ ARMS ❏ SHOULDERS ❏ BACK ❏ LEGS ❏ CORE

STRENGTH						
EXERCISE	SET 1		SET 2		SET 3	
	Reps	Weight	Reps	Weight	Reps	Weight

CARDIO					
EXERCISE	Duration	km/mi	Speed	Incline	Calories

TOTAL LENGTH OF WORKOUT SESSION: _____MINUTES

MACRONUTRIENTS				
CARBS	FATS	PROTEINS	SODIUM	SUGARS

EVALUATION: ☆ ☆ ☆ ☆ ☆

SLEEP: _____HOURS   **WATER INTAKE:** _____oz/mL

FITNESS MYTH #5:

Exercising to Build Muscle Is the Best Way to Lose Weight

Do it for the gains (lift, that is). But if weight loss is the goal, weight lifting alone may not be the right exercise for you. Don't get me wrong, we all need to do curls for the guys and the girls. But weight lifting builds muscle mass, which, while it may take up less room on your body, is denser than fat. Because of this, weight lifting may not be the best path to weight loss.

When you are trying to lose weight, your primary goal should be to burn fat. And to burn fat, you must burn more calories than you digest. The question you should be asking yourself is: What exercises burn the most calories? When the Harvard Medical School compiled data on the calories burned by doing 30 minutes of various activities in 2004, they found that, among 20 common gym activities, general weight lifting burned the fewest calories—even less than activities like badminton, tai chi, gardening, and childcare. General weight lifting only burned more calories than extremely low-exertion activities like billiards, cooking, sitting in class, and sleeping. Vigorous weight lifting fared better, but weight lifting overall is low on the calorie-burning hierarchy.

Should you be lifting weights? Absolutely. Weight lifting builds and maintains muscles. If you are trying to lose weight, find something you enjoy doing that consumes a lot of calories, then supplement it with weight lifting. Think of weight loss as an upside-down pyramid: Diet covers the top 95% of the pyramid, calorie-burning activities account for 3% near the bottom, and weight lifting fills the last 2% at the tip. You've got to have curls for the guys and the girls!

DATE:_____ ❏ S ❏ M ❏ T ❏ W ❏ T ❏ F ❏ S

TODAY'S ACTIVITY:

❏ STRENGTH ❏ CARDIO ❏ OTHER_____

MUSCLE GROUP FOCUS:

❏ CHEST ❏ ARMS ❏ SHOULDERS ❏ BACK ❏ LEGS ❏ CORE

EXERCISE	STRENGTH					
	SET 1		SET 2		SET 3	
	Reps	Weight	Reps	Weight	Reps	Weight

CARDIO					
EXERCISE	Duration	km/mi	Speed	Incline	Calories

TOTAL LENGTH OF WORKOUT SESSION:_____MINUTES

MACRONUTRIENTS				
CARBS	FATS	PROTEINS	SODIUM	SUGARS

EVALUATION: ☆ ☆ ☆ ☆ ☆

SLEEP:_____HOURS   **WATER INTAKE:**_____oz/mL

DATE:_____   ❏ S ❏ M ❏ T ❏ W ❏ T ❏ F ❏ S

TODAY'S ACTIVITY:

❏ STRENGTH   ❏ CARDIO   ❏ OTHER _____

MUSCLE GROUP FOCUS:

❏ CHEST   ❏ ARMS   ❏ SHOULDERS   ❏ BACK   ❏ LEGS   ❏ CORE

STRENGTH						
EXERCISE	**SET 1**		**SET 2**		**SET 3**	
	Reps	Weight	Reps	Weight	Reps	Weight

CARDIO					
EXERCISE	Duration	km/mi	Speed	Incline	Calories

TOTAL LENGTH OF WORKOUT SESSION: _____MINUTES

MACRONUTRIENTS				
CARBS	**FATS**	**PROTEINS**	**SODIUM**	**SUGARS**

EVALUATION: ☆ ☆ ☆ ☆ ☆

SLEEP: _____HOURS   **WATER INTAKE:** _____oz/mL

DATE:_____ ❏ S ❏ M ❏ T ❏ W ❏ T ❏ F ❏ S

TODAY'S ACTIVITY:

❏ STRENGTH   ❏ CARDIO   ❏ OTHER _____

MUSCLE GROUP FOCUS:

❏ CHEST   ❏ ARMS   ❏ SHOULDERS   ❏ BACK   ❏ LEGS   ❏ CORE

	STRENGTH					
EXERCISE	**SET 1**		**SET 2**		**SET 3**	
	Reps	Weight	Reps	Weight	Reps	Weight

	CARDIO				
EXERCISE	Duration	km/mi	Speed	Incline	Calories

TOTAL LENGTH OF WORKOUT SESSION: _____MINUTES

MACRONUTRIENTS				
CARBS	**FATS**	**PROTEINS**	**SODIUM**	**SUGARS**

EVALUATION: ☆ ☆ ☆ ☆ ☆

SLEEP: _____HOURS   **WATER INTAKE:** _____oz/mL

DATE:_____   ❏ S ❏ M ❏ T ❏ W ❏ T ❏ F ❏ S

TODAY'S ACTIVITY:

❏ STRENGTH   ❏ CARDIO   ❏ OTHER _____

MUSCLE GROUP FOCUS:

❏ CHEST   ❏ ·ARMS   ❏ SHOULDERS   ❏ BACK   ❏ LEGS   ❏ CORE

EXERCISE	STRENGTH					
	SET 1		SET 2		SET 3	
	Reps	Weight	Reps	Weight	Reps	Weight

CARDIO					
EXERCISE	Duration	km/mi	Speed	Incline	Calories

TOTAL LENGTH OF WORKOUT SESSION: _____MINUTES

MACRONUTRIENTS				
CARBS	FATS	PROTEINS	SODIUM	SUGARS

EVALUATION: ☆ ☆ ☆ ☆ ☆

SLEEP: _____HOURS   **WATER INTAKE:** _____oz/mL

DATE:_____ ❑ S ❑ M ❑ T ❑ W ❑ T ❑ F ❑ S

TODAY'S ACTIVITY:

❑ STRENGTH ❑ CARDIO ❑ OTHER _____

MUSCLE GROUP FOCUS:

❑ CHEST ❑ ARMS ❑ SHOULDERS ❑ BACK ❑ LEGS ❑ CORE

STRENGTH						
EXERCISE	**SET 1**		**SET 2**		**SET 3**	
	Reps	Weight	Reps	Weight	Reps	Weight

CARDIO					
EXERCISE	Duration	km/mi	Speed	Incline	Calories

TOTAL LENGTH OF WORKOUT SESSION: _____ MINUTES

MACRONUTRIENTS				
CARBS	**FATS**	**PROTEINS**	**SODIUM**	**SUGARS**

EVALUATION: ☆ ☆ ☆ ☆ ☆

SLEEP: _____ HOURS **WATER INTAKE:** _____ oz/mL

DATE:_____ ❑ S ❑ M ❑ T ❑ W ❑ T ❑ F ❑ S

TODAY'S ACTIVITY:

❑ STRENGTH   ❑ CARDIO   ❑ OTHER _____

MUSCLE GROUP FOCUS:

❑ CHEST   ❑ ARMS   ❑ SHOULDERS   ❑ BACK   ❑ LEGS   ❑ CORE

STRENGTH						
EXERCISE	**SET 1**		**SET 2**		**SET 3**	
	Reps	Weight	Reps	Weight	Reps	Weight

CARDIO					
EXERCISE	Duration	km/mi	Speed	Incline	Calories

TOTAL LENGTH OF WORKOUT SESSION: _____MINUTES

MACRONUTRIENTS				
CARBS	**FATS**	**PROTEINS**	**SODIUM**	**SUGARS**

EVALUATION: ☆ ☆ ☆ ☆ ☆

SLEEP: _____HOURS   **WATER INTAKE:** _____oz/mL

DATE:＿＿＿＿＿＿＿＿ ❑ S ❑ M ❑ T ❑ W ❑ T ❑ F ❑ S

TODAY'S ACTIVITY:

❑ STRENGTH ❑ CARDIO ❑ OTHER＿＿＿＿＿＿＿＿＿＿

MUSCLE GROUP FOCUS:

❑ CHEST ❑ ARMS ❑ SHOULDERS ❑ BACK ❑ LEGS ❑ CORE

	STRENGTH					
EXERCISE	SET 1		SET 2		SET 3	
	Reps	Weight	Reps	Weight	Reps	Weight

CARDIO					
EXERCISE	Duration	km/mi	Speed	Incline	Calories

TOTAL LENGTH OF WORKOUT SESSION:＿＿＿＿＿＿＿MINUTES

MACRONUTRIENTS				
CARBS	FATS	PROTEINS	SODIUM	SUGARS

EVALUATION: ☆ ☆ ☆ ☆ ☆

SLEEP:＿＿＿＿＿HOURS **WATER INTAKE:**＿＿＿＿＿oz/mL

DATE:_____ ❑ S ❑ M ❑ T ❑ W ❑ T ❑ F ❑ S

TODAY'S ACTIVITY:

❑ STRENGTH   ❑ CARDIO   ❑ OTHER _____

MUSCLE GROUP FOCUS:

❑ CHEST   ❑ ARMS   ❑ SHOULDERS   ❑ BACK   ❑ LEGS   ❑ CORE

STRENGTH						
EXERCISE	**SET 1**		**SET 2**		**SET 3**	
	Reps	Weight	Reps	Weight	Reps	Weight

CARDIO					
EXERCISE	Duration	km/mi	Speed	Incline	Calories

TOTAL LENGTH OF WORKOUT SESSION: _____MINUTES

MACRONUTRIENTS				
CARBS	**FATS**	**PROTEINS**	**SODIUM**	**SUGARS**

EVALUATION: ☆ ☆ ☆ ☆ ☆

SLEEP: _____HOURS   **WATER INTAKE:** _____oz/mL

DATE:_____ ❑ S ❑ M ❑ T ❑ W ❑ T ❑ F ❑ S

TODAY'S ACTIVITY:

❑ STRENGTH ❑ CARDIO ❑ OTHER _____

MUSCLE GROUP FOCUS:

❑ CHEST ❑ ARMS ❑ SHOULDERS ❑ BACK ❑ LEGS ❑ CORE

| EXERCISE | STRENGTH | | | | | |
| | SET 1 | | SET 2 | | SET 3 | |
	Reps	Weight	Reps	Weight	Reps	Weight

| CARDIO | | | | | |
EXERCISE	Duration	km/mi	Speed	Incline	Calories

TOTAL LENGTH OF WORKOUT SESSION: _____MINUTES

| MACRONUTRIENTS | | | | |
CARBS	FATS	PROTEINS	SODIUM	SUGARS

EVALUATION: ☆ ☆ ☆ ☆ ☆

SLEEP: _____HOURS   **WATER INTAKE:** _____oz/mL

DATE:_____   ❏ S ❏ M ❏ T ❏ W ❏ T ❏ F ❏ S

TODAY'S ACTIVITY:

❏ STRENGTH   ❏ CARDIO   ❏ OTHER _____

MUSCLE GROUP FOCUS:

❏ CHEST   ❏ ARMS   ❏ SHOULDERS   ❏ BACK   ❏ LEGS   ❏ CORE

STRENGTH						
EXERCISE	**SET 1**		**SET 2**		**SET 3**	
	Reps	Weight	Reps	Weight	Reps	Weight

CARDIO					
EXERCISE	Duration	km/mi	Speed	Incline	Calories

TOTAL LENGTH OF WORKOUT SESSION: _____MINUTES

MACRONUTRIENTS				
CARBS	**FATS**	**PROTEINS**	**SODIUM**	**SUGARS**

EVALUATION: ☆ ☆ ☆ ☆ ☆

SLEEP: _____HOURS   **WATER INTAKE:** _____oz/mL

FITNESS MYTH #6:
If You're Not Sweating, You're Not Working

We all remember Rocky Balboa running up the steps of the Philadelphia Museum of Art in sweaty clothes and doing sweaty one-handed push-ups on the mat. Sweat means you're really losing weight, right? Not necessarily.

Sweat is your body's way of cooling itself down. We sweat to regulate our body temperature, and in doing so, we lose stored water. Upon rehydration, the lost water weight returns. The mere act of sweating during any workout is not a good barometer of the workout's effectiveness. Many factors contribute to sweating, such as age, weight, fitness level, medical conditions, hydration, alcohol consumption, stress, temperature, environment, and genetics.

According to research first presented in 2014 by Brian Tracy of Colorado State University, 90 minutes of infamously sweaty Bikram yoga performed in a room heated to 105 degrees Fahrenheit burns an average of 460 calories for men and 330 for women. That's roughly equivalent to the calories burned by walking briskly (at a speed of about 3.5 miles per hour) for 90 minutes—but such a walk conducted in cold weather would produce tremendously less sweat than hot yoga would. Sweat is not a reliable measurement of calories burned or weight lost.

How can you figure out how many calories you've burned during a workout? Try using tools like an activity tracker, a heart rate monitor, or a table listing metabolic equivalent of task (MET) thresholds. (MET is a unit used to estimate the amount of energy consumed by the body in physical activity.) Whichever method you choose, the most important thing is to track your calories burned!

MEASUREMENT LOG 3

DATE:_____

NECK	
CHEST	
SHOULDER WIDTH	
RIGHT UPPER ARM	
LEFT UPPER ARM	
RIGHT FOREARM	
LEFT FOREARM	
WAIST	
HIPS	
RIGHT THIGH	
LEFT THIGH	
RIGHT CALF	
LEFT CALF	
BMI	
RMR	
RHR	

DATE:_____ ❑ S ❑ M ❑ T ❑ W ❑ T ❑ F ❑ S

TODAY'S ACTIVITY:

❑ STRENGTH   ❑ CARDIO   ❑ OTHER _____

MUSCLE GROUP FOCUS:

❑ CHEST   ❑ ARMS   ❑ SHOULDERS   ❑ BACK   ❑ LEGS   ❑ CORE

STRENGTH						
EXERCISE	SET 1		SET 2		SET 3	
	Reps	Weight	Reps	Weight	Reps	Weight

CARDIO					
EXERCISE	Duration	km/mi	Speed	Incline	Calories

TOTAL LENGTH OF WORKOUT SESSION: _____MINUTES

MACRONUTRIENTS				
CARBS	FATS	PROTEINS	SODIUM	SUGARS

EVALUATION: ☆ ☆ ☆ ☆ ☆

SLEEP: _____HOURS   **WATER INTAKE:** _____oz/mL

DATE:_____ ❑ S ❑ M ❑ T ❑ W ❑ T ❑ F ❑ S

TODAY'S ACTIVITY:

❑ STRENGTH ❑ CARDIO ❑ OTHER _____

MUSCLE GROUP FOCUS:

❑ CHEST ❑ ARMS ❑ SHOULDERS ❑ BACK ❑ LEGS ❑ CORE

STRENGTH						
EXERCISE	SET 1		SET 2		SET 3	
	Reps	Weight	Reps	Weight	Reps	Weight

CARDIO					
EXERCISE	Duration	km/mi	Speed	Incline	Calories

TOTAL LENGTH OF WORKOUT SESSION: _____MINUTES

MACRONUTRIENTS				
CARBS	FATS	PROTEINS	SODIUM	SUGARS

EVALUATION: ☆ ☆ ☆ ☆ ☆

SLEEP: _____HOURS **WATER INTAKE:** _____oz/mL

DATE:_____ ❑ S ❑ M ❑ T ❑ W ❑ T ❑ F ❑ S

TODAY'S ACTIVITY:

❑ STRENGTH   ❑ CARDIO   ❑ OTHER _____

MUSCLE GROUP FOCUS:

❑ CHEST   ❑ ARMS   ❑ SHOULDERS   ❑ BACK   ❑ LEGS   ❑ CORE

	STRENGTH						
EXERCISE	SET 1		SET 2		SET 3		
	Reps	Weight	Reps	Weight	Reps	Weight	

	CARDIO				
EXERCISE	Duration	km/mi	Speed	Incline	Calories

TOTAL LENGTH OF WORKOUT SESSION: _____ MINUTES

MACRONUTRIENTS					
CARBS	**FATS**	**PROTEINS**	**SODIUM**	**SUGARS**	

EVALUATION: ☆ ☆ ☆ ☆ ☆

SLEEP: _____ HOURS   **WATER INTAKE:** _____ oz/mL

DATE:_____ ❑ S ❑ M ❑ T ❑ W ❑ T ❑ F ❑ S

TODAY'S ACTIVITY:

❑ STRENGTH   ❑ CARDIO   ❑ OTHER _____

MUSCLE GROUP FOCUS:

❑ CHEST   ❑ ARMS   ❑ SHOULDERS   ❑ BACK   ❑ LEGS   ❑ CORE

STRENGTH						
EXERCISE	**SET 1**		**SET 2**		**SET 3**	
	Reps	Weight	Reps	Weight	Reps	Weight

CARDIO					
EXERCISE	Duration	km/mi	Speed	Incline	Calories

TOTAL LENGTH OF WORKOUT SESSION: _____MINUTES

MACRONUTRIENTS				
CARBS	**FATS**	**PROTEINS**	**SODIUM**	**SUGARS**

EVALUATION: ☆ ☆ ☆ ☆ ☆

SLEEP: _____HOURS   **WATER INTAKE:** _____oz/mL

DATE:_____ ❏ S ❏ M ❏ T ❏ W ❏ T ❏ F ❏ S

TODAY'S ACTIVITY:

❏ STRENGTH ❏ CARDIO ❏ OTHER _____

MUSCLE GROUP FOCUS:

❏ CHEST ❏ ARMS ❏ SHOULDERS ❏ BACK ❏ LEGS ❏ CORE

STRENGTH						
EXERCISE	**SET 1**		**SET 2**		**SET 3**	
	Reps	Weight	Reps	Weight	Reps	Weight

CARDIO					
EXERCISE	Duration	km/mi	Speed	Incline	Calories

TOTAL LENGTH OF WORKOUT SESSION: _____MINUTES

MACRONUTRIENTS				
CARBS	**FATS**	**PROTEINS**	**SODIUM**	**SUGARS**

EVALUATION: ☆ ☆ ☆ ☆ ☆

SLEEP: _____HOURS   **WATER INTAKE:** _____oz/mL

DATE:_____   ❏ S   ❏ M   ❏ T   ❏ W   ❏ T   ❏ F   ❏ S

TODAY'S ACTIVITY:

❏ STRENGTH   ❏ CARDIO   ❏ OTHER _____

MUSCLE GROUP FOCUS:

❏ CHEST   ❏ ARMS   ❏ SHOULDERS   ❏ BACK   ❏ LEGS   ❏ CORE

STRENGTH						
EXERCISE	**SET 1**		**SET 2**		**SET 3**	
	Reps	Weight	Reps	Weight	Reps	Weight

CARDIO					
EXERCISE	Duration	km/mi	Speed	Incline	Calories

TOTAL LENGTH OF WORKOUT SESSION: _____MINUTES

MACRONUTRIENTS				
CARBS	**FATS**	**PROTEINS**	**SODIUM**	**SUGARS**

EVALUATION: ☆ ☆ ☆ ☆ ☆

SLEEP: _____HOURS   **WATER INTAKE:** _____oz/mL

DATE:_____   ❏ S ❏ M ❏ T ❏ W ❏ T ❏ F ❏ S

TODAY'S ACTIVITY:

❏ STRENGTH   ❏ CARDIO   ❏ OTHER _____

MUSCLE GROUP FOCUS:

❏ CHEST   ❏ ARMS   ❏ SHOULDERS   ❏ BACK   ❏ LEGS   ❏ CORE

STRENGTH						
EXERCISE	**SET 1**		**SET 2**		**SET 3**	
	Reps	Weight	Reps	Weight	Reps	Weight

CARDIO					
EXERCISE	Duration	km/mi	Speed	Incline	Calories

TOTAL LENGTH OF WORKOUT SESSION: _____MINUTES

MACRONUTRIENTS				
CARBS	**FATS**	**PROTEINS**	**SODIUM**	**SUGARS**

EVALUATION: ☆ ☆ ☆ ☆ ☆

SLEEP: _____HOURS   **WATER INTAKE:** _____oz/mL

DATE:_____ ❑ S ❑ M ❑ T ❑ W ❑ T ❑ F ❑ S

TODAY'S ACTIVITY:

❑ STRENGTH ❑ CARDIO ❑ OTHER _____

MUSCLE GROUP FOCUS:

❑ CHEST ❑ ARMS ❑ SHOULDERS ❑ BACK ❑ LEGS ❑ CORE

EXERCISE	STRENGTH					
	SET 1		SET 2		SET 3	
	Reps	Weight	Reps	Weight	Reps	Weight

CARDIO					
EXERCISE	Duration	km/mi	Speed	Incline	Calories

TOTAL LENGTH OF WORKOUT SESSION: _____ MINUTES

MACRONUTRIENTS				
CARBS	FATS	PROTEINS	SODIUM	SUGARS

EVALUATION: ☆ ☆ ☆ ☆ ☆

SLEEP: _____ HOURS **WATER INTAKE:** _____ oz/mL

DATE:_____ ❏ S ❏ M ❏ T ❏ W ❏ T ❏ F ❏ S

TODAY'S ACTIVITY:

❏ STRENGTH ❏ CARDIO ❏ OTHER _____

MUSCLE GROUP FOCUS:

❏ CHEST ❏ ARMS ❏ SHOULDERS ❏ BACK ❏ LEGS ❏ CORE

	STRENGTH					
EXERCISE	**SET 1**		**SET 2**		**SET 3**	
	Reps	Weight	Reps	Weight	Reps	Weight

	CARDIO				
EXERCISE	Duration	km/mi	Speed	Incline	Calories

TOTAL LENGTH OF WORKOUT SESSION: _____ MINUTES

MACRONUTRIENTS				
CARBS	**FATS**	**PROTEINS**	**SODIUM**	**SUGARS**

EVALUATION: ☆ ☆ ☆ ☆ ☆

SLEEP: _____ HOURS **WATER INTAKE:** _____ oz/mL

DATE:_____   ❏ S   ❏ M   ❏ T   ❏ W   ❏ T   ❏ F   ❏ S

TODAY'S ACTIVITY:

❏ STRENGTH   ❏ CARDIO   ❏ OTHER _____

MUSCLE GROUP FOCUS:

❏ CHEST   ❏ ARMS   ❏ SHOULDERS   ❏ BACK   ❏ LEGS   ❏ CORE

STRENGTH						
EXERCISE	SET 1		SET 2		SET 3	
	Reps	Weight	Reps	Weight	Reps	Weight

CARDIO					
EXERCISE	Duration	km/mi	Speed	Incline	Calories

TOTAL LENGTH OF WORKOUT SESSION: _____MINUTES

MACRONUTRIENTS				
CARBS	FATS	PROTEINS	SODIUM	SUGARS

EVALUATION: ☆ ☆ ☆ ☆ ☆

SLEEP: _____HOURS   **WATER INTAKE:** _____oz/mL

Tracking Your Progress Doesn't Matter

How can we know who we are and where we are going if we don't know anything about where we have come from and what we have been through, the courage shown, the costs paid, to be where we are?

—David McCullough

The mind is a funny thing. The randomness of which memories stick and which do not always astounds me. I have been on this weight-loss journey for three years now. Some days I forget what life was like at 475 pounds. I forget about being unable to tie my shoes or get in and out of a vehicle. David McCullough is right. We need to remember the courage we've shown and the costs we've paid to get where we are in life.

You are undergoing a 90-day transformation. Recording and tracking everything in this journal will keep you on point and disciplined. The information you write down will be invaluable in determining the next step of your fitness journey. And most important, this journal will provide the before-and-after records that will keep you from backtracking. Knowing where you came from will prevent you from repeating history.

If I ever start slipping, I can look back at my 475-pound pictures and remember the misery. There is no going back for me. Poet and author Maya Angelou said it most succinctly: "You can't really know where you are going until you know where you have been." Get to journaling, boys!

DATE:_____   ❑ S ❑ M ❑ T ❑ W ❑ T ❑ F ❑ S

TODAY'S ACTIVITY:

❑ STRENGTH   ❑ CARDIO   ❑ OTHER _____

MUSCLE GROUP FOCUS:

❑ CHEST   ❑ ARMS   ❑ SHOULDERS   ❑ BACK   ❑ LEGS   ❑ CORE

EXERCISE	STRENGTH					
	SET 1		SET 2		SET 3	
	Reps	Weight	Reps	Weight	Reps	Weight

EXERCISE	CARDIO				
	Duration	km/mi	Speed	Incline	Calories

TOTAL LENGTH OF WORKOUT SESSION: _____MINUTES

MACRONUTRIENTS				
CARBS	FATS	PROTEINS	SODIUM	SUGARS

EVALUATION: ☆ ☆ ☆ ☆ ☆

SLEEP: _____HOURS   **WATER INTAKE:** _____oz/mL

DATE:_____   ❏ S ❏ M ❏ T ❏ W ❏ T ❏ F ❏ S

TODAY'S ACTIVITY:

❏ STRENGTH   ❏ CARDIO   ❏ OTHER _____

MUSCLE GROUP FOCUS:

❏ CHEST   ❏ ARMS   ❏ SHOULDERS   ❏ BACK   ❏ LEGS   ❏ CORE

STRENGTH						
EXERCISE	**SET 1**		**SET 2**		**SET 3**	
	Reps	Weight	Reps	Weight	Reps	Weight

CARDIO					
EXERCISE	Duration	km/mi	Speed	Incline	Calories

TOTAL LENGTH OF WORKOUT SESSION: _____MINUTES

MACRONUTRIENTS				
CARBS	**FATS**	**PROTEINS**	**SODIUM**	**SUGARS**

EVALUATION: ☆ ☆ ☆ ☆ ☆

SLEEP: _____HOURS   **WATER INTAKE:** _____oz/mL

DATE:_____ ❏ S ❏ M ❏ T ❏ W ❏ T ❏ F ❏ S

TODAY'S ACTIVITY:

❏ STRENGTH   ❏ CARDIO   ❏ OTHER _____

MUSCLE GROUP FOCUS:

❏ CHEST   ❏ ARMS   ❏ SHOULDERS   ❏ BACK   ❏ LEGS   ❏ CORE

STRENGTH						
EXERCISE	**SET 1**		**SET 2**		**SET 3**	
	Reps	Weight	Reps	Weight	Reps	Weight

CARDIO					
EXERCISE	Duration	km/mi	Speed	Incline	Calories

TOTAL LENGTH OF WORKOUT SESSION: _____MINUTES

MACRONUTRIENTS				
CARBS	**FATS**	**PROTEINS**	**SODIUM**	**SUGARS**

EVALUATION: ☆ ☆ ☆ ☆ ☆

SLEEP: _____HOURS   **WATER INTAKE:** _____oz/mL

DATE:_____   ❏ S ❏ M ❏ T ❏ W ❏ T ❏ F ❏ S

TODAY'S ACTIVITY:

❏ STRENGTH   ❏ CARDIO   ❏ OTHER _____

MUSCLE GROUP FOCUS:

❏ CHEST   ❏ ARMS   ❏ SHOULDERS   ❏ BACK   ❏ LEGS   ❏ CORE

STRENGTH						
EXERCISE	**SET 1**		**SET 2**		**SET 3**	
	Reps	Weight	Reps	Weight	Reps	Weight

CARDIO					
EXERCISE	Duration	km/mi	Speed	Incline	Calories

TOTAL LENGTH OF WORKOUT SESSION: _____MINUTES

MACRONUTRIENTS				
CARBS	**FATS**	**PROTEINS**	**SODIUM**	**SUGARS**

EVALUATION: ☆ ☆ ☆ ☆ ☆

SLEEP: _____HOURS   **WATER INTAKE:** _____oz/mL

DATE:_____   ❏ S ❏ M ❏ T ❏ W ❏ T ❏ F ❏ S

TODAY'S ACTIVITY:

❏ STRENGTH   ❏ CARDIO   ❏ OTHER _____

MUSCLE GROUP FOCUS:

❏ CHEST   ❏ ARMS   ❏ SHOULDERS   ❏ BACK   ❏ LEGS   ❏ CORE

EXERCISE	STRENGTH					
	SET 1		SET 2		SET 3	
	Reps	Weight	Reps	Weight	Reps	Weight

CARDIO					
EXERCISE	Duration	km/mi	Speed	Incline	Calories

TOTAL LENGTH OF WORKOUT SESSION: _____MINUTES

MACRONUTRIENTS				
CARBS	FATS	PROTEINS	SODIUM	SUGARS

EVALUATION: ☆ ☆ ☆ ☆ ☆

SLEEP: _____HOURS   **WATER INTAKE:** _____oz/mL

DATE:_____ ❑ S ❑ M ❑ T ❑ W ❑ T ❑ F ❑ S

TODAY'S ACTIVITY:

❑ STRENGTH   ❑ CARDIO   ❑ OTHER _____

MUSCLE GROUP FOCUS:

❑ CHEST   ❑ ARMS   ❑ SHOULDERS   ❑ BACK   ❑ LEGS   ❑ CORE

	STRENGTH						
EXERCISE	**SET 1**		**SET 2**		**SET 3**		
	Reps	Weight	Reps	Weight	Reps	Weight	

CARDIO					
EXERCISE	Duration	km/mi	Speed	Incline	Calories

TOTAL LENGTH OF WORKOUT SESSION: _____MINUTES

MACRONUTRIENTS				
CARBS	**FATS**	**PROTEINS**	**SODIUM**	**SUGARS**

EVALUATION: ☆ ☆ ☆ ☆ ☆

SLEEP: _____HOURS   **WATER INTAKE:** _____oz/mL

DATE:_____ ❏ S ❏ M ❏ T ❏ W ❏ T ❏ F ❏ S

TODAY'S ACTIVITY:

❏ STRENGTH   ❏ CARDIO   ❏ OTHER_____

MUSCLE GROUP FOCUS:

❏ CHEST   ❏ ARMS   ❏ SHOULDERS   ❏ BACK   ❏ LEGS   ❏ CORE

EXERCISE	STRENGTH					
	SET 1		SET 2		SET 3	
	Reps	Weight	Reps	Weight	Reps	Weight

CARDIO					
EXERCISE	Duration	km/mi	Speed	Incline	Calories

TOTAL LENGTH OF WORKOUT SESSION: _____MINUTES

MACRONUTRIENTS				
CARBS	**FATS**	**PROTEINS**	**SODIUM**	**SUGARS**

EVALUATION: ☆ ☆ ☆ ☆ ☆

SLEEP: _____HOURS   **WATER INTAKE:** _____oz/mL

DATE:_____   ❑ S ❑ M ❑ T ❑ W ❑ T ❑ F ❑ S

TODAY'S ACTIVITY:

❑ STRENGTH   ❑ CARDIO   ❑ OTHER _____

MUSCLE GROUP FOCUS:

❑ CHEST   ❑ ARMS   ❑ SHOULDERS   ❑ BACK   ❑ LEGS   ❑ CORE

STRENGTH						
EXERCISE	**SET 1**		**SET 2**		**SET 3**	
	Reps	Weight	Reps	Weight	Reps	Weight

CARDIO					
EXERCISE	Duration	km/mi	Speed	Incline	Calories

TOTAL LENGTH OF WORKOUT SESSION: _____MINUTES

MACRONUTRIENTS				
CARBS	**FATS**	**PROTEINS**	**SODIUM**	**SUGARS**

EVALUATION: ☆ ☆ ☆ ☆ ☆

SLEEP: _____HOURS   **WATER INTAKE:** _____oz/mL

DATE:_____ ❏ S ❏ M ❏ T ❏ W ❏ T ❏ F ❏ S

TODAY'S ACTIVITY:

❏ STRENGTH ❏ CARDIO ❏ OTHER _____

MUSCLE GROUP FOCUS:

❏ CHEST ❏ ARMS ❏ SHOULDERS ❏ BACK ❏ LEGS ❏ CORE

STRENGTH						
EXERCISE	**SET 1**		**SET 2**		**SET 3**	
	Reps	Weight	Reps	Weight	Reps	Weight

CARDIO					
EXERCISE	Duration	km/mi	Speed	Incline	Calories

TOTAL LENGTH OF WORKOUT SESSION: _____MINUTES

MACRONUTRIENTS				
CARBS	**FATS**	**PROTEINS**	**SODIUM**	**SUGARS**

EVALUATION: ☆ ☆ ☆ ☆ ☆

SLEEP: _____HOURS   **WATER INTAKE:** _____oz/mL

DATE:_____   ❏ S ❏ M ❏ T ❏ W ❏ T ❏ F ❏ S

TODAY'S ACTIVITY:

❏ STRENGTH   ❏ CARDIO   ❏ OTHER _____

MUSCLE GROUP FOCUS:

❏ CHEST   ❏ ARMS   ❏ SHOULDERS   ❏ BACK   ❏ LEGS   ❏ CORE

	STRENGTH					
EXERCISE	**SET 1**		**SET 2**		**SET 3**	
	Reps	Weight	Reps	Weight	Reps	Weight

CARDIO					
EXERCISE	Duration	km/mi	Speed	Incline	Calories

TOTAL LENGTH OF WORKOUT SESSION: _____ MINUTES

MACRONUTRIENTS				
CARBS	**FATS**	**PROTEINS**	**SODIUM**	**SUGARS**

EVALUATION: ☆ ☆ ☆ ☆ ☆

SLEEP: _____ HOURS   **WATER INTAKE:** _____ oz/mL

FITNESS MYTH #8:
Hours Spent Sleeping Are Irrelevant

Time is the least thing we have of.
—Ernest Hemingway

There is never enough time in the day. As a result, sleep often suffers first. If your goal is to lose weight, a good night's sleep should be your top priority. The Harvard T.H. Chan School of Public Health surveyed dozens of studies on the relationship between sleep and obesity and determined most of them suggested a correlation between lack of sleep and increased weight. One study from New Zealand found that every one-hour reduction in sleep during childhood was connected with a 50 percent increase in risk of obesity at age 32. That is crazy.

Another example from the Harvard survey: The longest and largest study of adult sleep and weight to date is the Nurses' Health Study, which, over the course of three cohorts, has followed hundreds of thousands of American women for decades. Analyzing the first cohort, which was established in 1976, researchers found that women who slept 5 hours a night were 15 percent more likely to become obese than those who slept 7 hours a night.

The Harvard survey concludes: "There is convincing evidence that getting a less than ideal amount of sleep is an independent and strong risk factor for obesity, in infants and children as well as in adults." I can't encourage you enough to read this article (see References, page 116) and to get your butt in bed!

MEASUREMENT LOG 4

DATE:_____

NECK		
CHEST		
SHOULDER WIDTH		
RIGHT UPPER ARM		
LEFT UPPER ARM		
RIGHT FOREARM		
LEFT FOREARM		
WAIST		
HIPS		
RIGHT THIGH		
LEFT THIGH		
RIGHT CALF		
LEFT CALF		
BMI		
RMR		
RHR		

DATE:_____ ❏ S ❏ M ❏ T ❏ W ❏ T ❏ F ❏ S

TODAY'S ACTIVITY:

❏ STRENGTH   ❏ CARDIO   ❏ OTHER _____

MUSCLE GROUP FOCUS:

❏ CHEST   ❏ ARMS   ❏ SHOULDERS   ❏ BACK   ❏ LEGS   ❏ CORE

STRENGTH					
EXERCISE	**SET 1**		**SET 2**		**SET 3**	
	Reps	Weight	Reps	Weight	Reps	Weight

CARDIO					
EXERCISE	Duration	km/mi	Speed	Incline	Calories

TOTAL LENGTH OF WORKOUT SESSION: _____ MINUTES

MACRONUTRIENTS				
CARBS	**FATS**	**PROTEINS**	**SODIUM**	**SUGARS**

EVALUATION: ☆ ☆ ☆ ☆ ☆

SLEEP: _____ HOURS   **WATER INTAKE:** _____ oz/mL

DATE:_____   ❑ S ❑ M ❑ T ❑ W ❑ T ❑ F ❑ S

TODAY'S ACTIVITY:

❑ STRENGTH   ❑ CARDIO   ❑ OTHER _____

MUSCLE GROUP FOCUS:

❑ CHEST   ❑ ARMS   ❑ SHOULDERS   ❑ BACK   ❑ LEGS   ❑ CORE

STRENGTH					
EXERCISE	SET 1		SET 2		SET 3	
	Reps	Weight	Reps	Weight	Reps	Weight

CARDIO					
EXERCISE	Duration	km/mi	Speed	Incline	Calories

TOTAL LENGTH OF WORKOUT SESSION: _____MINUTES

MACRONUTRIENTS				
CARBS	FATS	PROTEINS	SODIUM	SUGARS

EVALUATION: ☆ ☆ ☆ ☆ ☆

SLEEP: _____HOURS   **WATER INTAKE:** _____oz/mL

DATE:_____ ❑ S ❑ M ❑ T ❑ W ❑ T ❑ F ❑ S

TODAY'S ACTIVITY:

❑ STRENGTH ❑ CARDIO ❑ OTHER _____

MUSCLE GROUP FOCUS:

❑ CHEST ❑ ARMS ❑ SHOULDERS ❑ BACK ❑ LEGS ❑ CORE

EXERCISE	SET 1		SET 2		SET 3	
	Reps	Weight	Reps	Weight	Reps	Weight

STRENGTH

EXERCISE	Duration	km/mi	Speed	Incline	Calories

CARDIO

TOTAL LENGTH OF WORKOUT SESSION: _____ MINUTES

CARBS	FATS	PROTEINS	SODIUM	SUGARS

MACRONUTRIENTS

EVALUATION: ☆ ☆ ☆ ☆ ☆

SLEEP: _____ HOURS   **WATER INTAKE:** _____ oz/mL

DATE:_____ ❑ S ❑ M ❑ T ❑ W ❑ T ❑ F ❑ S

TODAY'S ACTIVITY:

❑ STRENGTH   ❑ CARDIO   ❑ OTHER _____

MUSCLE GROUP FOCUS:

❑ CHEST   ❑ ARMS   ❑ SHOULDERS   ❑ BACK   ❑ LEGS   ❑ CORE

STRENGTH						
EXERCISE	SET 1		SET 2		SET 3	
	Reps	Weight	Reps	Weight	Reps	Weight

CARDIO					
EXERCISE	Duration	km/mi	Speed	Incline	Calories

TOTAL LENGTH OF WORKOUT SESSION: _____MINUTES

MACRONUTRIENTS				
CARBS	FATS	PROTEINS	SODIUM	SUGARS

EVALUATION: ☆ ☆ ☆ ☆ ☆

SLEEP: _____HOURS   **WATER INTAKE:** _____oz/mL

DATE:_____   ❑ S ❑ M ❑ T ❑ W ❑ T ❑ F ❑ S

TODAY'S ACTIVITY:

❑ STRENGTH   ❑ CARDIO   ❑ OTHER _____

MUSCLE GROUP FOCUS:

❑ CHEST   ❑ ARMS   ❑ SHOULDERS   ❑ BACK   ❑ LEGS   ❑ CORE

EXERCISE	STRENGTH					
	SET 1		SET 2		SET 3	
	Reps	Weight	Reps	Weight	Reps	Weight

CARDIO					
EXERCISE	Duration	km/mi	Speed	Incline	Calories

TOTAL LENGTH OF WORKOUT SESSION: _____MINUTES

MACRONUTRIENTS				
CARBS	FATS	PROTEINS	SODIUM	SUGARS

EVALUATION: ☆ ☆ ☆ ☆ ☆

SLEEP: _____HOURS   **WATER INTAKE:** _____oz/mL

DATE:_____ ❑ S ❑ M ❑ T ❑ W ❑ T ❑ F ❑ S

TODAY'S ACTIVITY:

❑ STRENGTH ❑ CARDIO ❑ OTHER_____

MUSCLE GROUP FOCUS:

❑ CHEST ❑ ARMS ❑ SHOULDERS ❑ BACK ❑ LEGS ❑ CORE

EXERCISE	STRENGTH					
	SET 1		SET 2		SET 3	
	Reps	Weight	Reps	Weight	Reps	Weight

EXERCISE	CARDIO				
	Duration	km/mi	Speed	Incline	Calories

TOTAL LENGTH OF WORKOUT SESSION:_____MINUTES

MACRONUTRIENTS				
CARBS	FATS	PROTEINS	SODIUM	SUGARS

EVALUATION: ☆ ☆ ☆ ☆ ☆

SLEEP:_____HOURS **WATER INTAKE:**_____oz/mL

DATE:_____   ❏ S ❏ M ❏ T ❏ W ❏ T ❏ F ❏ S

TODAY'S ACTIVITY:

❏ STRENGTH   ❏ CARDIO   ❏ OTHER_____

MUSCLE GROUP FOCUS:

❏ CHEST   ❏ ARMS   ❏ SHOULDERS   ❏ BACK   ❏ LEGS   ❏ CORE

EXERCISE	STRENGTH					
	SET 1		SET 2		SET 3	
	Reps	Weight	Reps	Weight	Reps	Weight

CARDIO					
EXERCISE	Duration	km/mi	Speed	Incline	Calories

TOTAL LENGTH OF WORKOUT SESSION: _____MINUTES

MACRONUTRIENTS				
CARBS	FATS	PROTEINS	SODIUM	SUGARS

EVALUATION: ☆ ☆ ☆ ☆ ☆

SLEEP: _____HOURS   **WATER INTAKE:** _____oz/mL

DATE:_____   ❑ S   ❑ M   ❑ T   ❑ W   ❑ T   ❑ F   ❑ S

TODAY'S ACTIVITY:

❑ STRENGTH   ❑ CARDIO   ❑ OTHER _____

MUSCLE GROUP FOCUS:

❑ CHEST   ❑ ARMS   ❑ SHOULDERS   ❑ BACK   ❑ LEGS   ❑ CORE

STRENGTH							
EXERCISE		SET 1		SET 2		SET 3	
		Reps	Weight	Reps	Weight	Reps	Weight

CARDIO					
EXERCISE	Duration	km/mi	Speed	Incline	Calories

TOTAL LENGTH OF WORKOUT SESSION: _____ MINUTES

MACRONUTRIENTS				
CARBS	FATS	PROTEINS	SODIUM	SUGARS

EVALUATION: ☆ ☆ ☆ ☆ ☆

SLEEP: _____ HOURS   **WATER INTAKE:** _____ oz/mL

DATE:_____ ❑ S ❑ M ❑ T ❑ W ❑ T ❑ F ❑ S

TODAY'S ACTIVITY:
❑ STRENGTH   ❑ CARDIO   ❑ OTHER _____

MUSCLE GROUP FOCUS:
❑ CHEST   ❑ ARMS   ❑ SHOULDERS   ❑ BACK   ❑ LEGS   ❑ CORE

STRENGTH						
EXERCISE	SET 1		SET 2		SET 3	
	Reps	Weight	Reps	Weight	Reps	Weight

CARDIO					
EXERCISE	Duration	km/mi	Speed	Incline	Calories

TOTAL LENGTH OF WORKOUT SESSION: _____MINUTES

MACRONUTRIENTS				
CARBS	FATS	PROTEINS	SODIUM	SUGARS

EVALUATION: ☆ ☆ ☆ ☆ ☆

SLEEP: _____HOURS   **WATER INTAKE:** _____oz/mL

DATE:_____ ❑ S ❑ M ❑ T ❑ W ❑ T ❑ F ❑ S

TODAY'S ACTIVITY:

❑ STRENGTH ❑ CARDIO ❑ OTHER _____

MUSCLE GROUP FOCUS:

❑ CHEST ❑ ARMS ❑ SHOULDERS ❑ BACK ❑ LEGS ❑ CORE

	STRENGTH						
	EXERCISE	SET 1		SET 2		SET 3	
		Reps	Weight	Reps	Weight	Reps	Weight

CARDIO					
EXERCISE	Duration	km/mi	Speed	Incline	Calories

TOTAL LENGTH OF WORKOUT SESSION: _____MINUTES

MACRONUTRIENTS					
CARBS	FATS	PROTEINS	SODIUM	SUGARS	

EVALUATION: ☆ ☆ ☆ ☆ ☆

SLEEP: _____HOURS **WATER INTAKE:** _____oz/mL

FITNESS MYTH #9:
You Shouldn't Reward Yourself

The highest reward for a person's toil is not what they get for it, but what they become by it.

—John Ruskin

The greatest reward of your fitness journey will be the new you. In 90 days, you will lose weight, gain muscle, develop healthy habits, and achieve greater mental focus. Your life will change, and you will want to push yourself even further. Nothing will top the feeling of the new you. Yet all work and no play makes Jack a dull boy.

Rewarding yourself is an essential part of the journey. Rewards give you something to work for and look forward to while you put in the hours at the gym or on the mat. Make your rewards something special, but make sure they won't derail your fitness plans. Your reward of choice could be a weekend getaway, a massage, new clothes, new toys, time alone, fishing—whatever is important to you.

You might observe that I did not mention food in that list of rewards. If you can reward yourself with non-diet food and return immediately to losing weight, then food rewards are okay. I can't. Once I eat certain foods, I can't stop eating them. I know that I am one bite away from 475 pounds. Make your reward something you can control, not an excuse to feed your addiction.

Reward yourself. You deserve it. Just don't make the reward part of the poison. Have fun, and lighten up, Jack!

PART III

REVIEW RESULTS

You did it! Ninety days in the books. Awesome job!

Regardless of whether you worked out religiously or intermittently, you are here, still reading, writing, and striving for a better life. Nothing is better than that. For 90 days, you maintained your goal to be healthy. This journal is the record of your hard work, dedication, sweat, and accomplishments. No one can take that away from you.

This is your history and scorecard. Review its pages and your progress. Notice how the food you ate evolved, the workouts developed, the measurements changed, and your mental attitude shifted. All of this is hard data. Use it to plot your course for the next 90 days. Now you have information specific to you, and you know what works and what doesn't. Think about your journey, buy a new journal, and let's keep this train moving forward!

LESSONS LEARNED

Change is inevitable but personal growth is a choice.
—Bob Proctor

It is time to study the data and extract its lessons. Look unflinchingly on your journey and choose your next course of action.

Your Inner Journey

On this page, I want you to reflect on your weight-loss experience. I know it's not easy to dig deep. But exercise affects you mentally just as much as it does physically. What have you learned about yourself by chronicling this journey? What would you tell "you" from 90 days ago? Capture that here.

_____

_____

_____

_____

_____

_____

_____

_____

_____

_____

_____

_____

_____

Your Outer Journey

While you have achieved much, the journey doesn't end here. As you observe your outer body and newfound strength and flexibility, think of where you want to go from here. Write down three goals for the next 90 days. Once you put them to paper, they have power—so the more specific, the better. I want to know exactly where you plan to be in three months.

_____

_____

_____

_____

_____

_____

_____

_____

_____

_____

_____

_____

_____

_____

_____

_____

MEASUREMENT LOG: RESULTS

Congratulations! It's your final Measurement Log! These results are your final scorecard and the starting point for the next 90 days.

DATE:_____

NECK	
CHEST	
SHOULDER WIDTH	
RIGHT UPPER ARM	
LEFT UPPER ARM	
RIGHT FOREARM	
LEFT FOREARM	
WAIST	
HIPS	
RIGHT THIGH	
LEFT THIGH	
RIGHT CALF	
LEFT CALF	
BMI	
RMR	
RHR	

RESOURCES

Listed here are books, websites, and an app that played key roles in my weight-loss journey and can help you in yours.

BOOKS

Discipline Equals Freedom: Field Manual, by Jocko Willink

The Obesity Code: Unlocking the Secrets of Weight Loss, by Jason Fung

Positively Unstoppable: The Art of Owning It, by Diamond Dallas Page

Smarter Workouts: The Science of Exercise Made Simple, by Pete McCall

WEBSITES

ButcherBox, *ButcherBox.com*

CDC BMI Calculator, *CDC.gov/healthyweight/assessing/bmi/adult_bmi/english_bmi_calculator/bmi_calculator.html*

DDP Yoga (DDPY), *DDPYoga.com*

DDP Yoga Facebook Group, *Facebook.com/groups/ddpyoga*

DDPY Nutrition, *Guide-DDPYoga.com/nutrition*

Healthy Eater Flexible Dieting Macro Calculator, *HealthyEater.com/flexible-dieting-calculator*

MyFitnessPal BMR Calculator, *MyFitnessPal.com/tools/bmr-calculator*

WebMD Food Calculator, *WebMD.com/diet/healthtool-food-calorie-counter*

APP

MyFitnessPal

REFERENCES

Ainsworth, Barbara E., William L. Haskell, Stephen D. Herrmann, Nathanael Meckes, David R. Bassett Jr., Catrine Tudor-Locke, Jennifer L. Greer, Jesse Vezina, Melicia C. Whitt-Glover, Arthur S. Leon. "Compendium of Physical Activities: A Second Update of Codes and MET Values." *Medicine and Science in Sports and Exercise* 43, no. 8 (August 2011): 1575–1581.

Blackburn, Kellie Bramlet. "How to Determine Calorie Burn." *MD Anderson Cancer Center Focused on Health* (blog), June 2017. MDAnderson.org/publications /focused-on-health/How-to-determine-calorie-burn.h27Z1591413.html.

"Calories Burned in 30 Minutes for People of Three Different Weights." *Harvard Heart Letter. Harvard Health Publishing.* Last modified August 13, 2018. health.harvard.edu/diet-and-weight-loss/calories-burned-in-30-minutes -of-leisure-and-routine-activities.

Dodge, Jeff. "Researcher: 'Hot' Yoga Yields Fitness Benefits." *Colorado State University Source* (blog), July 15, 2014. source.colostate.edu/researcher -hot-yoga-yields-fitness-benefits.

Gunnars, Kris. "How Many Calories Should You Eat per Day to Lose Weight?" *Healthline* (blog), December 19, 2019. healthline.com/nutrition /how-many-calories-per-day.

Harvard T. H. Chan School of Public Health. "Obesity Prevention Source: Sleep." Accessed September 27, 2020. https://www.hsph.harvard.edu /obesity-prevention-source/obesity-causes/sleep-and-obesity.

La Berge, Ann F. "How the Ideology of Low Fat Conquered America." *Journal of the History of Medicine and Allied Sciences* 63, no. 2 (February 2008): 139–177.

Lally, Philippa, Cornelia H. M. van Jaarsveld, Henry W. W. Potts, and Jane Wardle. "How Are Habits Formed: Modelling Habit Formation in the Real World." *European Journal of Social Psychology* 40 (July 2010): 998–1009.

McMurray, Robert G., Jesus Soares, Carl J. Caspersen, Thomas McCurdy. "Examining Variations of Resting Metabolic Rate of Adults: A Public Health Perspective." *Medicine and Science in Sports and Exercise* 46, no. 7 (July 2014): 1352–1358.

ACKNOWLEDGMENTS

I must start by thanking my wife, Mary. Thank you for believing in and sticking with me. I could not have done this without you. I also want to thank my editors, Joe Cho and Andrea Leptinsky, and the whole team at Rockridge Press. I could not have written this book without your guidance and support.

Thank you to comedian Bert Kreischer. Bert's running of the St. Pete Half Marathon was the starting point of my journey. And thank you to Steve Yu, President of DDP Yoga. Steve changed my life with his video of my story.

Lastly, I have to thank the man himself, Diamond Dallas Page. Dallas gave me a second life. Thank you so much for creating DDPY, reaching out to me on Twitter, and staying on me daily. You are right, Dallas: "You can own your life!" Thank you, Dallas, for everything.

ABOUT THE AUTHOR

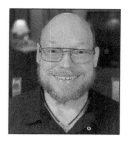

Vance Hinds is a husband to a beautiful wife of 30 years, and father to three beautiful, independent, grown children. After losing 198 pounds in 12 months with diet and exercise alone, Vance has maintained the weight loss for over 3 years. Vance is a career attorney, a DDP Yoga fanatic, and the creator of two podcasts, *Extrausual* and *1K Ton Goal*.

Vance's goal is to bring hope to the hopeless and help others in similar situations. As Vance's mentor Diamond Dallas Page says: "You can own your life!" Vance's current mission is to inspire 10,000 people to lose 200 pounds each, removing 1,000 tons of body weight from this planet. To be part of the 1K Ton Goal Project, visit 1KTon.com.